# Depression

Editor: Danielle Lobban

Volume 404

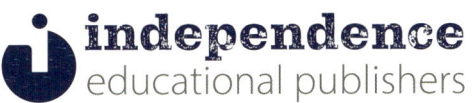

First published by Independence Educational Publishers

The Studio, High Green

Great Shelford

Cambridge CB22 5EG

England

© Independence 2022

## Copyright

This book is sold subject to the condition that it shall not,
by way of trade or otherwise, be lent, resold, hired out or otherwise
circulated in any form of binding or cover other than that in which it
is published without the publisher's prior consent.

## Photocopy licence

The material in this book is protected by copyright. However, the
purchaser is free to make multiple copies of particular articles for instructional
purposes for immediate use within the purchasing institution.
Making copies of the entire book is not permitted.

ISBN-13: 978 1 86168 863 7

## Printed in Great Britain

Zenith Print Group

# Contents

## Chapter 1: About Depression

| | |
|---|---|
| Types of depression | 1 |
| Depression | 2 |
| Postnatal depression | 4 |
| Coronavirus and depression in adults, Great Britain: July to August 2021 | 6 |
| The difference between burnout and depression | 8 |
| Depression and anxiety rose sharply over Christmas in the UK | 11 |
| People with depression can sometimes experience memory problems – here's why | 12 |
| A changing brain: how depression can alter our brain structure | 14 |
| Night owls more likely to be depressed because they have to work against their natural body clock, says study | 17 |
| Does depression exist? | 18 |
| 'Overlooked and underfunded': experts call for global action to deal with depression | 20 |

## Chapter 2: Coping & Therapies

| | |
|---|---|
| | 21 |
| Piecing life back together after a period of depression | 23 |
| NHS to give therapy for depression before medication under new guidelines | 27 |
| Ketamine therapy swiftly reduces depression and suicidal thoughts | 28 |
| A world without antidepressants: the new alternatives to prescription pills | 29 |
| Mark Cavendish keen to use his battle with depression to help others | 31 |
| Best evidence suggests antidepressants aren't very effective in kids and teens. What can be done instead? | 32 |
| You can't control the headlines but here's some stuff you can control | 33 |
| How to cope with bad news | 34 |
| Talking therapies | 36 |

| | |
|---|---|
| Key Facts | 40 |
| Glossary | 41 |
| Activities | 42 |
| Index | 43 |
| Acknowledgements | 44 |

# Introduction

Depression is Volume 404 in the **issues** series. The aim of the series is to offer current, diverse information about important issues in our world, from a UK perspective.

### About Depression

One in four of the population is affected by depression. It can happen to anyone at any time in their life. Globally the pandemic has had a huge impact on people's mental health with reports and diagnoses of depression rising steadily since 2020. This book looks at the different types of depression and both established and experimental treatments for it. It also considers the causes and symptoms of depression and ways to support those we know who may be afflicted.

### OUR SOURCES

Titles in the **issues** series are designed to function as educational resource books, providing a balanced overview of a specific subject.

The information in our books is comprised of facts, articles and opinions from many different sources, including:

- Newspaper reports and opinion pieces
- Website factsheets
- Magazine and journal articles
- Statistics and surveys
- Government reports
- Literature from special interest groups.

### A NOTE ON CRITICAL EVALUATION

Because the information reprinted here is from a number of different sources, readers should bear in mind the origin of the text and whether the source is likely to have a particular bias when presenting information (or when conducting their research). It is hoped that, as you read about the many aspects of the issues explored in this book, you will critically evaluate the information presented.

It is important that you decide whether you are being presented with facts or opinions. Does the writer give a biased or unbiased report? If an opinion is being expressed, do you agree with the writer? Is there potential bias to the 'facts' or statistics behind an article?

### ASSIGNMENTS

In the back of this book, you will find a selection of assignments designed to help you engage with the articles you have been reading and to explore your own opinions. Some tasks will take longer than others and there is a mixture of design, writing and research-based activities that you can complete alone or in a group.

### FURTHER RESEARCH

At the end of each article we have listed its source and a website that you can visit if you would like to conduct your own research. Please remember to critically evaluate any sources that you consult and consider whether the information you are viewing is accurate and unbiased.

## Useful Websites

www.blurtitout.org

www.independent.co.uk

www.mentalhealth.org.uk

www.mentalhealthtoday.co.uk

www.mentalhealth-uk.org

www.metro.co.uk

www.ons.gov.uk

www.positive.news

www.telegraph.co.uk

www.thecalmzone.net

www.theconversation.com

www.theguardian.com

www.ucl.ac.uk

www.unherd.com

www.who.int

# Chapter 1: About Depression

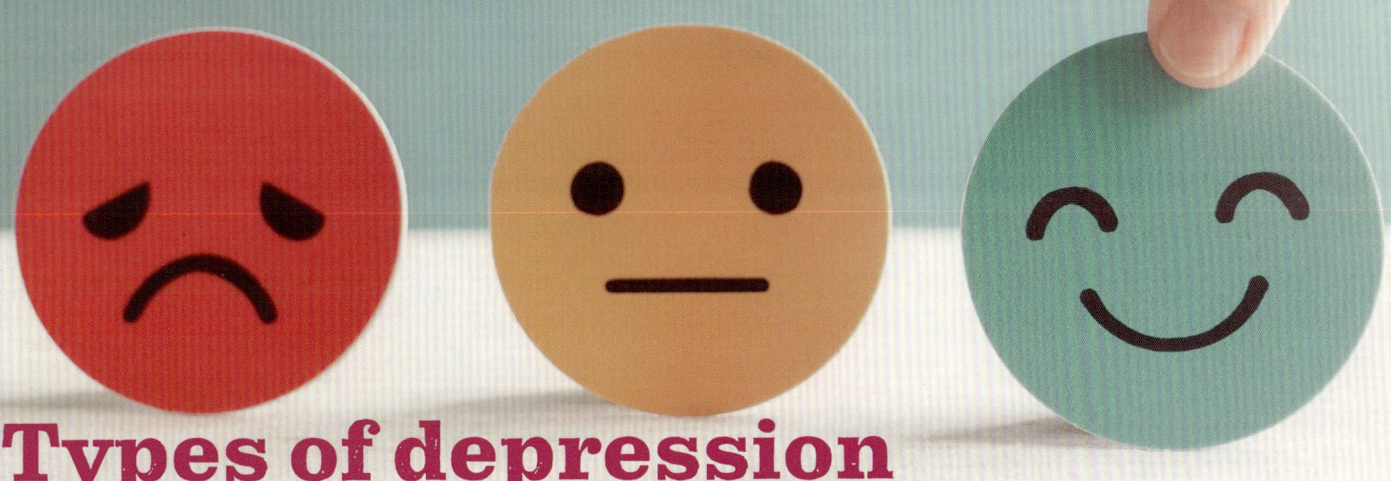

# Types of depression

## There are many different types of depression

### Clinical depression
Clinical depression means that a doctor has given you a diagnosis of depression.

### Depressive episode
This is the formal name that doctors give depression when they make a diagnosis. They may say that you're going through a 'mild', 'moderate' or 'severe' episode.

### Recurrent depressive disorder
If you've had at least 2 depressive episodes, your doctor might say that you have a recurrent depressive disorder. They may say that your current 'episode' is 'mild', 'moderate' or 'severe'.

### Reactive depression
If your doctor thinks that your depression was triggered by difficult events in your life, such as divorce or money worries, they may say that it is reactive.

### Dysthymia
This is when you are experiencing continuous mild depression that lasts for over 2 years. Also sometimes called persistent depressive disorder or chronic depression.

### Cyclothymia
You may be diagnosed with cyclothymia if you experience persistent and unstable moods. You may have periods of depression and periods of elation, but these periods may not be severe enough or long enough to be diagnosed as bipolar disorder.

### Manic depression
Manic depression is the name doctors used to use for bipolar disorder. It is not the same illness as depression, but people with bipolar disorder experience periods of depression as well as periods of extreme highs.

### Psychotic depression
If you experience a severe episode of depression, you may get hallucinations or delusions. These symptoms are called psychosis. A hallucination means you might hear, see, smell, taste or feel things that aren't real. A delusion means that you might believe things that don't match reality.

### Prenatal or postnatal depression
Prenatal depression occurs during pregnancy, it may also be called antenatal depression.

Postnatal depression occurs after becoming a parent. It can affect both men and women.

### Seasonal affective disorder (SAD)
If you have SAD, you'll experience depression during particular seasons, or because of certain types of weather. You might find that your mood or energy levels drop when it gets colder or warmer, or notice changes in your sleeping or eating patterns.

It will affect you at the same time of year every year. It's most common during the winter.

*2022*

The above information is reprinted with kind permission from Mental Health UK
© Mental Health UK

www.mentalhealth-uk.org

# Depression

## Key facts

- Depression is a common mental disorder. Globally, it is estimated that 5.0% of adults suffer from depression[1].
- Depression is a leading cause of disability worldwide and is a major contributor to the overall global burden of disease.
- More women are affected by depression than men.
- Depression can lead to suicide.
- There is effective treatment for mild, moderate, and severe depression.

## Overview

Depression is a common illness worldwide, with an estimated 3.8% of the population affected, including 5.0% among adults and 5.7% among adults older than 60 years[1]. Approximately 280 million people in the world have depression[1]. Depression is different from usual mood fluctuations and short-lived emotional responses to challenges in everyday life. Especially when recurrent and with moderate or severe intensity, depression may become a serious health condition. It can cause the affected person to suffer greatly and function poorly at work, at school and in the family. At its worst, depression can lead to suicide. Over 700 000 people die due to suicide every year. Suicide is the fourth leading cause of death in 15-29-year-olds.

Although there are known, effective treatments for mental disorders, more than 75% of people in low- and middle-income countries receive no treatment[2]. Barriers to effective care include a lack of resources, lack of trained health-care providers and social stigma associated with mental disorders. In countries of all income levels, people who experience depression are often not correctly diagnosed, and others who do not have the disorder are too often misdiagnosed and prescribed antidepressants.

### Symptoms and patterns

During a depressive episode, the person experiences depressed mood (feeling sad, irritable, empty) or a loss of pleasure or interest in activities, for most of the day, nearly every day, for at least two weeks. Several other symptoms are also present, which may include poor concentration, feelings of excessive guilt or low self-worth, hopelessness about the future, thoughts about dying or suicide, disrupted sleep, changes in appetite or weight, and feeling especially tired or low in energy.

In some cultural contexts, some people may express their mood changes more readily in the form of bodily symptoms (e.g. pain, fatigue, weakness). Yet, these physical symptoms are not due to another medical condition.

During a depressive episode, the person experiences significant difficulty in personal, family, social, educational, occupational, and/or other important areas of functioning.

A depressive episode can be categorised as mild, moderate, or severe depending on the number and severity of symptoms, as well as the impact on the individual's functioning.

### There are different patterns of mood disorders including:

- single episode depressive disorder, meaning the person's first and only episode);
- recurrent depressive disorder, meaning the person has a history of at least two depressive episodes; and

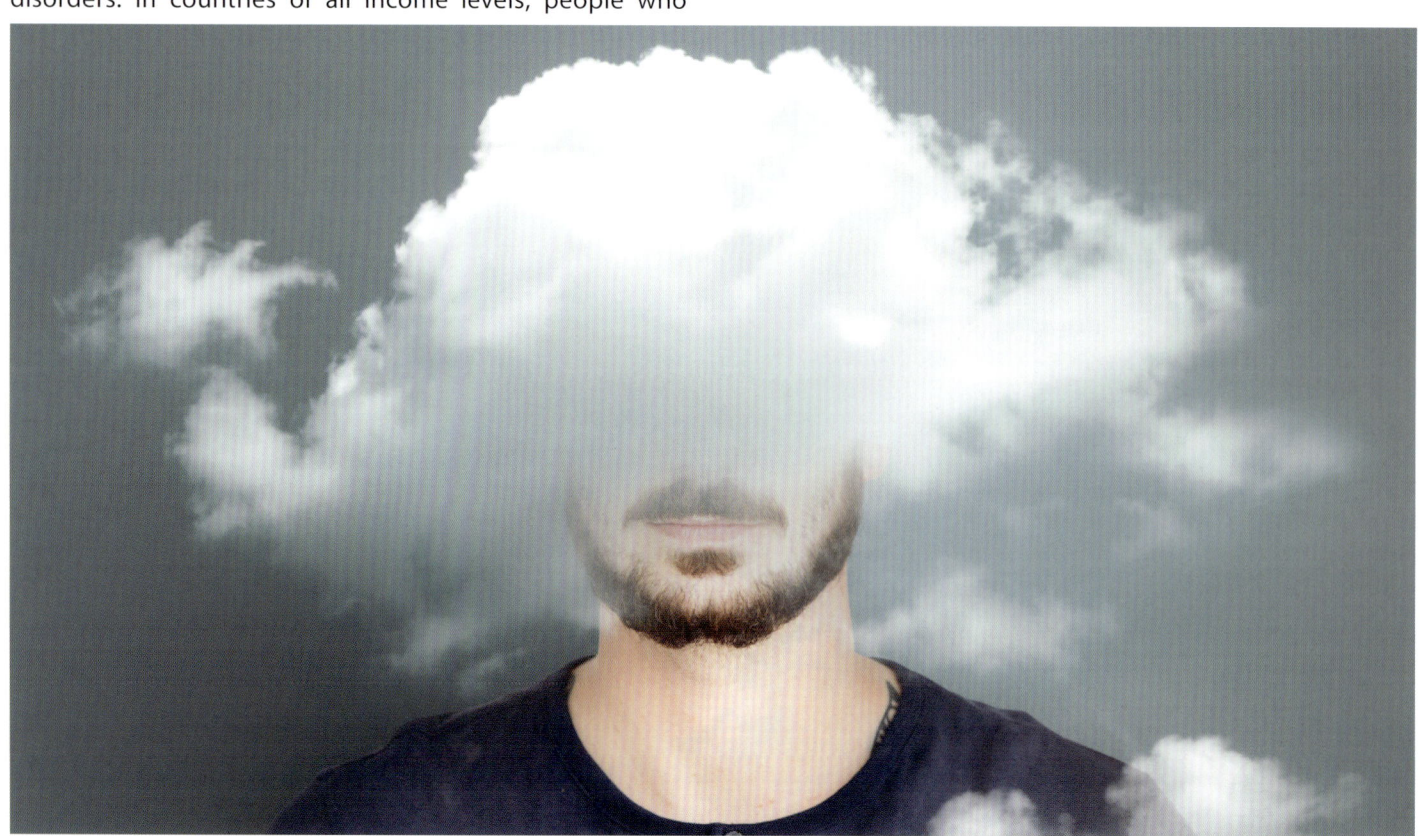

- bipolar disorder, meaning that depressive episodes alternate with periods of manic symptoms, which include euphoria or irritability, increased activity or energy, and other symptoms such as increased talkativeness, racing thoughts, increased self-esteem, decreased need for sleep, distractibility, and impulsive reckless behaviour.

## Contributing factors and prevention

Depression results from a complex interaction of social, psychological, and biological factors. People who have gone through adverse life events (unemployment, bereavement, traumatic events) are more likely to develop depression. Depression can, in turn, lead to more stress and dysfunction and worsen the affected person's life situation and the depression itself.

There are interrelationships between depression and physical health. For example, cardiovascular disease can lead to depression and vice versa.

Prevention programmes have been shown to reduce depression. Effective community approaches to prevent depression include school-based programmes to enhance a pattern of positive coping in children and adolescents. Interventions for parents of children with behavioural problems may reduce parental depressive symptoms and improve outcomes for their children. Exercise programmes for older persons can also be effective in depression prevention.

## Diagnosis and treatment

There are effective treatments for depression.

Depending on the severity and pattern of depressive episodes over time, health-care providers may offer psychological treatments such as behavioural activation, cognitive behavioural therapy and interpersonal psychotherapy, and/or antidepressant medication such as selective serotonin reuptake inhibitors (SSRIs) and tricyclic antidepressants (TCAs). Different medications are used for bipolar disorder. Health-care providers should keep in mind the possible adverse effects associated with antidepressant medication, the ability to deliver either intervention (in terms of expertise, and/or treatment availability), and individual preferences. Different psychological treatment formats for consideration include individual and/or group face-to-face psychological treatments delivered by professionals and supervised lay therapists. Antidepressants are not the first line of treatment for mild depression. They should not be used for treating depression in children and are not the first line of treatment in adolescents, among whom they should be used with extra caution.

## WHO response

WHO's Mental Health Action Plan 2013-2030 highlights the steps required to provide appropriate interventions for people with mental disorders including depression.

Depression is one of the priority conditions covered by WHO's Mental Health Gap Action Programme (mhGAP). The Programme aims to help countries increase services for people with mental, neurological and substance use disorders through care provided by health workers who are not specialists in mental health.

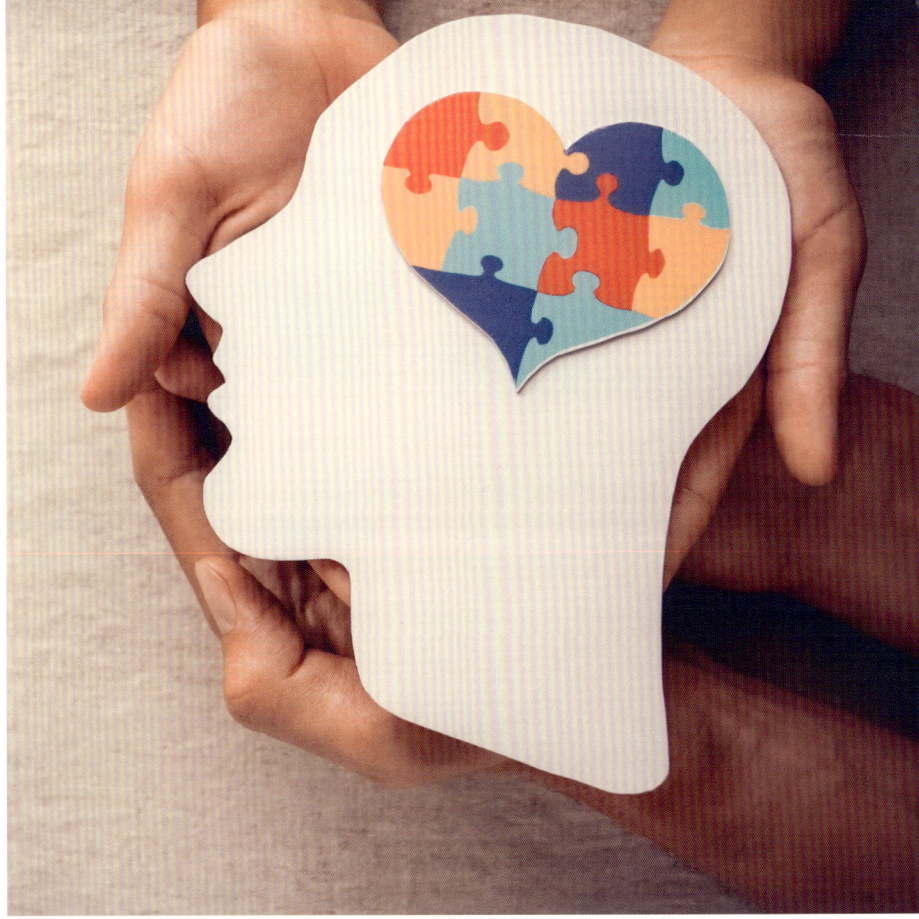

WHO has developed brief psychological intervention manuals for depression that may be delivered by lay workers to individuals and groups. An example is the Problem Management Plus manual, which describes the use of behavioural activation, stress management, problem solving treatment and strengthening social support. Moreover, the Group Interpersonal Therapy for Depression manual describes group treatment of depression. Finally, the Thinking Healthy manual covers the use of cognitive-behavioural therapy for perinatal depression.

References
1. Institute of Health Metrics and Evaluation. Global Health Data Exchange (GHDx). http://ghdx.healthdata.org/gbd-results-tool?params=gbd-api-2019- permalink/d780dffbe8a381b25e1416884959e88b (Accessed 1 May 2021).
2. Evans-Lacko S, Aguilar-Gaxiola S, Al-Hamzawi A, et al. Socio-economic variations in the mental health treatment gap for people with anxiety, mood, and substance use disorders: results from the WHO World Mental Health (WMH) surveys. Psychol Med. 2018;48(9):1560-1571.

*13 September 2021*

The above information is reprinted with kind permission from *World Health Organization*. © 2022 WHO

www.who.int/news-room/fact-sheets/detail/depression

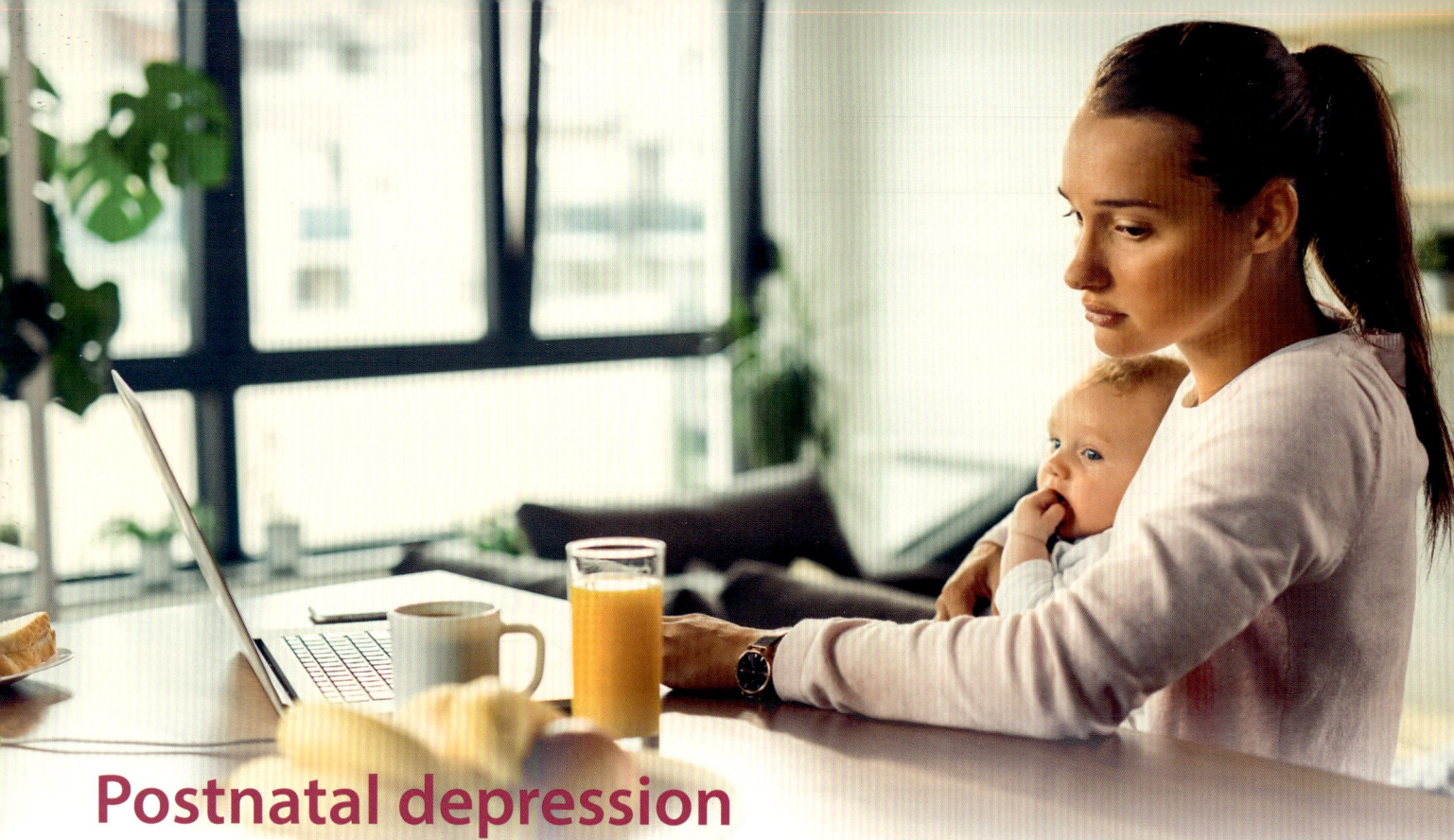

# Postnatal depression

Postnatal depression is a type of depression many people experience after having a baby. It's not the same as the 'baby blues': it needs treatment so you can recover.

Having a baby is a huge life event. It's normal to experience a range of powerful emotions while you're pregnant and after giving birth: excitement, joy, anxiety. You may also feel depressed. It's not a sign of weakness or anything to feel guilty about. With support and treatment, you can get better.

While most people have heard of postnatal depression, it's also possible to experience antenatal depression while you're pregnant. Some people experience both. The term 'perinatal depression' covers depression any time from getting pregnant to around a year after giving birth.

We've used the term 'postnatal depression' on this page as it's more well known, but the symptoms and treatment for antenatal or perinatal depression are the same.

## What is postnatal depression?

The 'baby blues' is a brief period of feeling low, emotional and tearful after giving birth. It doesn't last for more than two weeks of giving birth.

If your symptoms last longer or start later, you could have postnatal depression. It can start any time in the year after giving birth, and may begin gradually or suddenly. It can range from mild to severe.

It might be difficult to talk about how you're feeling. You may feel people expect you to be happy, or worry you're a bad parent if you tell someone you're depressed. Remember that postnatal depression can happen to anyone and isn't your fault. It's never too early or late to get help.

### What are the symptoms?

The symptoms of postnatal depression are similar to the symptoms of depression. They include:

♦ feeling sad or low

♦ being unable to enjoy things that normally bring you pleasure

♦ tiredness or loss in energy

♦ poor concentration or attention span

♦ low self-esteem and self-confidence

♦ disturbed sleep, even when your baby is asleep

♦ changes in appetite.

You may feel detached from your baby or partner. You may even have thoughts of hurting yourself or your baby. It can be very frightening to have thoughts of harming your baby, but remember this doesn't mean you're actually going to hurt them. The sooner you can talk to someone about your thoughts and feelings – a friend, relative, doctor or midwife, for instance – the sooner you can get the help you need.

### Can partners have postnatal depression?

Only people who have given birth in the last year can be formally diagnosed with postnatal depression, but evidence suggests partners can also experience anxiety or depression. This is a huge life change for them too, and dealing with a lack of sleep, extra household responsibilities and financial worries, for example, can be very difficult.

There is help and support available, either through their GP or specialist organisations such as the National Childbirth Trust, the Fatherhood Institute or PANDAS.

## What causes postnatal depression?

There are many reasons why someone can develop postnatal depression. These include:

- previous mental health problems
- hormonal changes during and after pregnancy
- your circumstances: for example, a lack of social support, stressful living conditions, losing your job, bereavement
- childhood experiences such as abuse, neglect or trauma. These may make it hard for you to relate to others, including your baby, or doubt your own parenting skills
- domestic violence or other abuse
- low self-esteem.

For many people, a combination of factors causes postnatal depression.

If you've experienced mental health problems in the past, tell your GP, health visitor and/or midwife. They can support you during and after pregnancy.

## Getting support

Being depressed doesn't mean you're a bad parent or that you're going mad. Some people worry it will mean their baby will be taken away from them. Remember that asking for help means you're doing the best for your baby: it's good parenting. Healthcare professionals will want to support you so you can look after your baby. Children are only taken into care in very exceptional circumstances.

If you have symptoms of postnatal depression, speak to your GP, health visitor and/or midwife. It's never too late to seek help: you can feel better even if you've had symptoms for a long time.

Different help is available depending on how severe your symptoms are.

### Talking therapy

You could be offered a self-help course or talking therapy such as Cognitive Behavioural Therapy (CBT). You can refer yourself for talking therapy in England.

CBT can help you see how the ways you think and behave may be making you feel depressed. For example, you may have unrealistic expectations about being a parent and feel you should never make a mistake. CBT can help you see these thoughts are unhelpful, and help you find a different way to think about parenthood.

### Medication

Antidepressants can help if your depression is severe or if talking therapy hasn't helped. If you're breastfeeding, your GP can recommend one that's safe to take.

### Specialist services

Specialist services are available if you need more support. These include:

- perinatal mental health services with specialist nurses and doctors who can help you get the right support
- community mental health teams (CMHTs). They can help if there aren't any perinatal mental health services in your area
- mother and baby units (MBUs). These are psychiatric wards in hospitals that can give you treatment and support as well as help you care for your baby. You'll have your own bedroom with a cot for your baby.

## Ways you can help yourself

Our page on depression has ideas on ways to look after yourself. As well as these, try to build a support network so you can meet friends and other new parents for a chat. Accept offers of help: don't feel you have to do everything yourself.

Tommy's has information about planning ahead for after the birth with practical tips on some of the practical and emotional stresses you may experience.

## What is postnatal psychosis?

Postnatal psychosis is a rare but serious illness. You may experience symptoms such as hearing or seeing things that aren't there, believing things that aren't true, mood swings, feeling confused and behaving in a way that is out of character. Symptoms usually start suddenly, often within hours or days of giving birth.

Postnatal psychosis (also known as postpartum psychosis) should be treated as a medical emergency. If you or your partner think you may have postnatal psychosis, seek medical help immediately from your GP, A&E or crisis team if you have one.

*Last updated: 18 February 2022*

### Useful resources

- The Association for Postnatal Illness can connect you to someone who has recovered from postnatal mental illness.
- Family Action and Family Rights Group both offer a range of practical and emotional support for parents.
- National Childbirth Trust offers information and support during pregnancy and early parenthood, including antenatal courses and local meet-ups.
- PANDAS offers support to anyone experiencing perinatal mental health problems. They have a helpline, support groups and tips on self-care.

The above information is reprinted with kind permission from the Mental Health Foundation
© 2022. All Rights Reserved

www.mentalhealth.org.uk

# Coronavirus and depression in adults, Great Britain: July to August 2021

Analysis of the proportion of the adult population of Great Britain experiencing some form of depression in summer 2021, based on the Opinions and Lifestyle Survey. Includes analysis by age, sex and other characteristics and comparisons with early 2021, 2020 and pre-pandemic estimates.

## Main points

- Around 1 in 6 (17%) adults experienced some form of depression in summer 2021 (21 July to 15 August); this is a decrease since early 2021 (21% during 27 January to 7 March) but is still above levels before the coronavirus (COVID-19) pandemic (10%).
- Rates of depressive symptoms peaked earlier in 2021 before falling to 17% at the end of March (31 March to 4 April); since then, levels have been largely stable.

Over the period 21 July to 15 August 2021:

- Younger adults and women were more likely to experience some form of depression, with around 1 in 3 (32%) women aged 16 to 29 years experiencing moderate to severe depressive symptoms, compared with 20% of men of the same age.
- Disabled (36%) and clinically extremely vulnerable (CEV) adults (28%) were more likely to experience some form of depression than non-disabled (8%) and non-CEV adults (16%).
- Around 3 in 10 (29%) adults who reported being unable to afford an unexpected expense of £850 experienced some form of depression, compared with around 1 in 10 (11%) adults who were able to afford this expense.
- Unemployed adults (31%) were twice as likely to experience some form of depression than those who were employed or self-employed (15%).
- Around 1 in 4 (24%) adults living in the most deprived areas of England experienced some form of depression; this compared with around 1 in 8 (12%) adults in the least deprived areas of England.
- Of adults experiencing some form of depression, almost three-quarters (74%) reported that the coronavirus pandemic was affecting their well-being; this compared with around one in three (32%) adults with no or mild depressive symptoms.

## Prevalence of depressive symptoms over time

Around one in six (17%) adults aged 16 years and over in Great Britain experienced some form of depression in summer 2021 (21 July to 15 August 2021). This is fewer than in early 2021 (27 January to 7 March 2021) (21%) and November 2020 (11 to 29 November 2020) (19%). However, rates in summer 2021 remained higher than those observed before the coronavirus (COVID-19) pandemic (July 2019 to March 2020), where 10% of adults experienced some form of depression (Figure 1).

**Figure 1: One in six adults experienced some form of depression in summer 2021, compared with one in five in early 2021**

Percentage of adults with moderate to severe depressive symptoms, Great Britain, July 2019 to August 2021

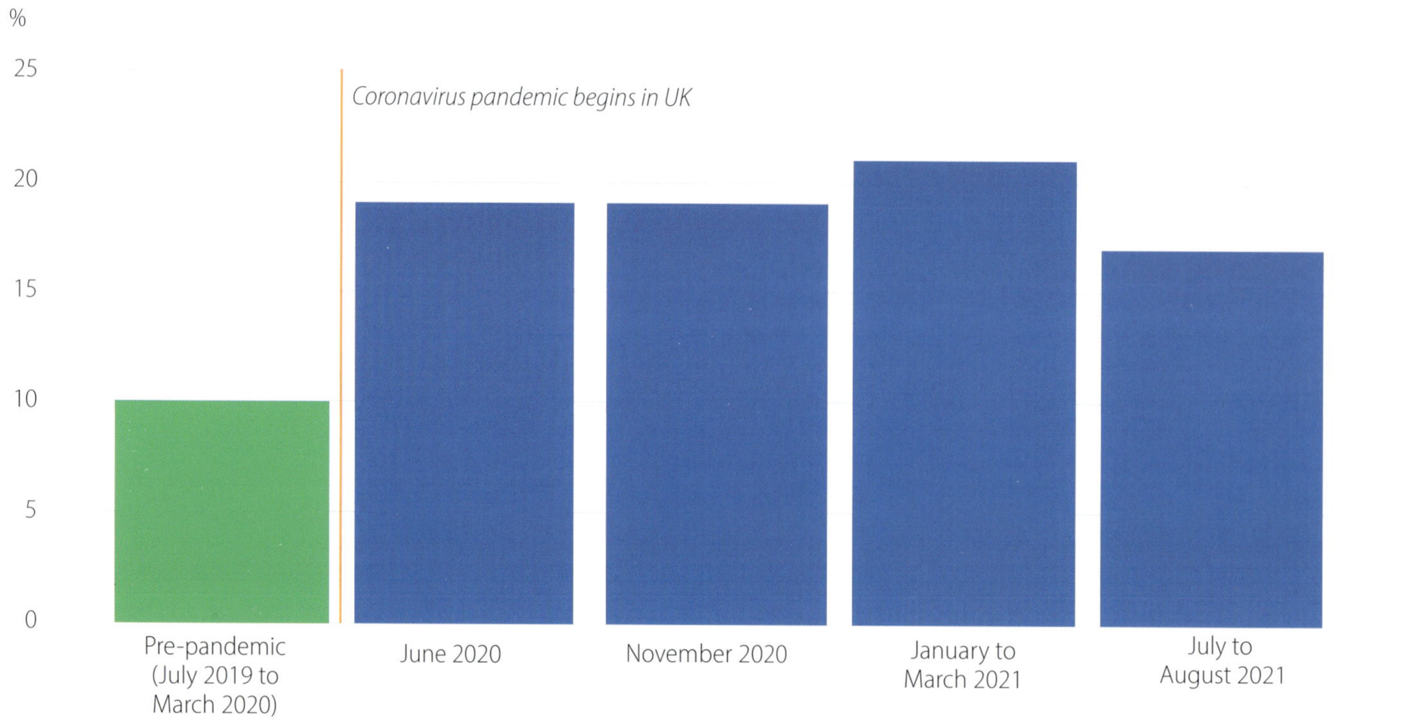

*Source: Office for National Statistics – Opinions and Lifestyle Survey*

## Figure 3: In summer 2021, rates of some form of depression declined across most population groups but remained higher than pre-pandemic levels

Percentage of adults with moderate to severe depressive symptoms, Great Britain, July 2019 to August 2021

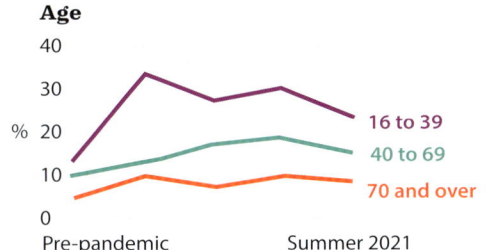
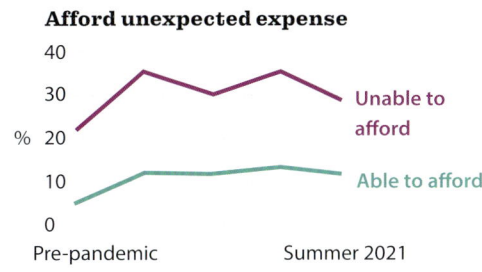
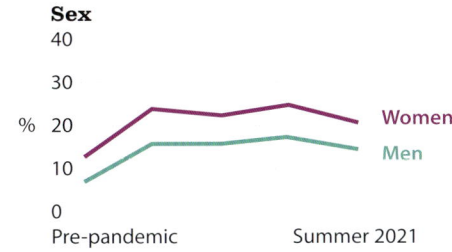
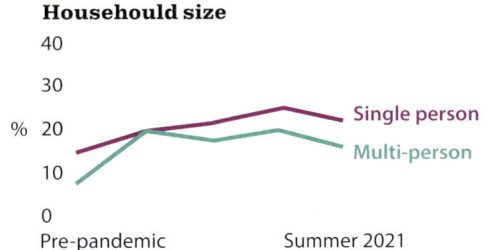
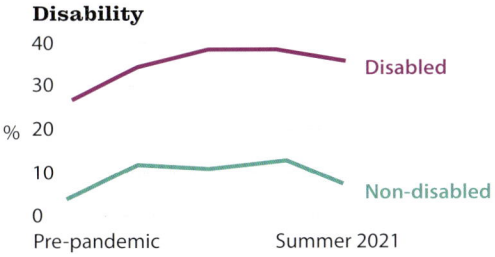
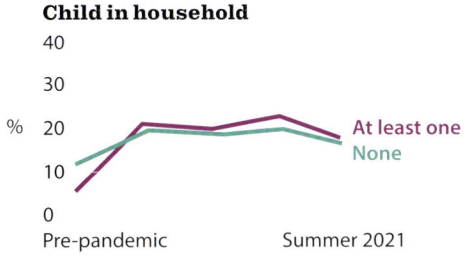

Source: Office for National Statistics – Opinions and Lifestyle Survey

The presence of some form of depression was indicated by a score of 10 or more on the eight-item Patient Health Questionnaire (PHQ8), which is also referred to as moderate to severe depressive symptoms. Further information can be found in the Glossary. Previous estimates of adults experiencing some form of depression using the same measure were published in August 2020, December 2020 and May 2021.

It is important to note that reasons for changes in the prevalence of depressive symptoms over time are likely to be complex. Reasons may include the impact of changes to restrictions related to the coronavirus pandemic and seasonal variation in levels of depressive symptoms, as well as other factors. As such, we cannot determine the cause of these changes from the analysis presented in this article.

### Comparison week-on-week

For the first time we have looked at weekly rates of adults experiencing some form of depression (indicated by moderate to severe depressive symptoms), covering the period 27 January to 22 August 2021.

Rates of moderate to severe depressive symptoms were highest earlier in the year before falling to 17% at the end of March (31 March to 4 April 2021). Since then, levels have been largely stable.

### Comparisons between population groups

Rates of some form of depression (indicated by moderate to severe depressive symptoms) in summer 2021 were lower across most population groups when compared to early 2021, although they remained higher than pre-pandemic levels. (Figure 3)

For adults aged 16 to 39 years, rates in summer 2021 were lower (23%) than early 2021 (29%) but were still more than double when compared with before the pandemic (11%). In comparison, the proportion of adults aged 70 years and over experiencing some form of depression remained stable between summer 2021 (9%) and early 2021 (10%), having increased from 5% before the pandemic.

In summer 2021, over one in four (29%) adults who reported being unable to afford an unexpected but necessary expense of £850 experienced some form of depression, having fallen from over one in three (35%) in early 2021. For adults who were able to afford this expense, 11% experienced moderate to severe depressive symptoms in summer 2021, decreasing from 13% in early 2021.

*1 October 2021*

The above information is reprinted with kind permission from the Office for National Statistics.
© Crown copyright 2021
This information is licensed under the Open Government Licence v3.0
To view this licence, visit http://www.nationalarchives.gov.uk/doc/open-government-licence/

www.ons.gov.uk

# The difference between burnout and depression

**B**urnout' is a term that people are becoming increasingly aware of. Many of the symptoms of burnout can be similar to those of depression and vice versa. Some people experience one but not the other, some find that one leads to the other and others experience both at the same time. It can be difficult to differentiate between the two.

## How common is burnout?

Though burnout can apply to different areas of life, it's most commonly spoken about in terms of work, so most statistics focus on work-related stress and burnout.

A 2020 survey revealed that around 22% of UK adults have experienced job-related burnout . In fact, in August 2020, over 27,000 people worldwide searched the term 'burnout symptoms'.

Google searches relating to burnout terms have increased over the last few years. However, whether burnout is more common, or whether more people are researching it because it's a term that's increasingly well-known, is currently unclear.

## What is burnout?

Burnout occurs when things have gone out of balance, and our stress and activity levels far outweigh the amount of rest we have.

Think about a fire. Fires need fuel, oxygen, and heat to burn. As it burns through fuel, there's less and less left to burn. If we add fuel to a fire, then it will continue to burn, but if we don't, it will eventually burn out. A burned-out fire has nothing left to give. It won't light and doesn't provide any heat. It's exhausted. To get it going again, we have to go back to the start, add more fuel, and re-light it.

As people, when we keep using up fuel (energy) without adding or recouping any, we eventually burn out. We don't have the energy we need to keep going.

## What does burnout feel like?

A key feature of burnout is exhaustion. We have a lack of energy and feel tired all the time.

Physically, we might catch more coughs and colds as our immune system dips. Our sleeping and eating habits might change. We might have frequent headaches.

Our alcohol consumption might increase, and if we smoke, we might be smoking more than usual. Sometimes we'll snap at others, have less patience, and become irritated or annoyed more quickly than normal. Over time, we might isolate ourselves from others and withdraw from our responsibilities.

We'll often feel negative about the situation our burnout relates to (eg. work or caring responsibilities) and might feel cynical and resentful. Our motivation, drive, and efficiency can all take a hit.

Sometimes, we turn the negativity we feel in on ourselves and view ourselves as a failure. We might feel annoyance or anger towards ourselves and blame ourselves for not being good enough (whatever 'good enough' means). Helplessness, loneliness and defeat can overwhelm us.

## Diagnosing burnout

Historically, there's been lots of debate over whether or not burnout can be classified as a medical condition.

Professionals have different opinions, and even diagnostic guides classify it differently. The World Health Organization officially recognised 'burn-out' as a 'syndrome' in 2019, but only in an occupational context. It will be included in the 11th edition of the International Classification of Diseases (ICD-11) which takes effect in January 2022. Despite this, it isn't currently included in the Diagnostic and Statistical Manual of Mental Disorders (DSM-5).

Even if clinicians are unable to diagnose burnout as a condition, they may still suggest that our experiences are due to long-term stress and/or exhaustion. Some may even use the term 'burnout' to describe our experiences.

## How do the causes of burnout and depression differ?

Burnout is often caused by excessive stress for a prolonged period. It's most commonly work-related, though some people think it's possible to experience burnout due to non-work situations, such as caring responsibilities, parenting, or wider family relationships.

It's often a gradual process and risk factors for experiencing burnout can include things like compassion fatigue, lack of recognition and reward, going a long time without a break, large amounts of pressure, unreasonable expectations, unmanageable workload, lack of control, lack of choice, and lack of autonomy.

Depression isn't usually caused by a single circumstance or event. Often, several different things will feed into it. Sometimes we won't be able to pinpoint anything specific at all. Some of the things that can contribute to depression include traumatic events, medical conditions, family circumstances, medication, culture, genetics, having a child, and family history.

## Burnout related to diagnosable conditions

Burnout can relate to specific situations and circumstances, such as work, but it's also increasingly being recognised as something which disproportionately affects people with some diagnosable conditions. For example, there's increasing evidence that autistic people, who've spent years 'masking', can experience autistic burnout. Some people think that there are also some links between burnout and Chronic Fatigue Syndrome (CFS), although they are not the same thing.

Though it's still related to high levels of stress and an imbalance of energy-out to energy-in, burnout related to other diagnosable conditions may differ slightly from work- or situation-specific burnout.

## How do symptoms of burnout and depression differ?

The key difference between burnout and depression is that burnout relates to a specific circumstance whereas depression is more generalised.

Where burnout can cause us to feel negatively towards a specific situation, depression may make us feel negative about lots of different things at once. Living with burnout can cause us to lose confidence in some of our abilities, depression can cause us to lose confidence in our ability to anything at all. Burnout might mean that we think we've failed at a specific 'thing'. But depression can cause us to feel as though we've failed as a person and failed at life.

The symptoms of the two can be similar, but the root causes are different, and as such the way to manage them can differ.

## How much does diagnosis matter?

People have different opinions on diagnosis, whatever the condition. Some view it as helpful, others don't.

Whichever name or label we choose to use (or not use), it can be helpful to try and work out whether there's a clear cause of our feelings, as that knowledge can aid our recovery.

Ultimately, choosing whether or not to investigate diagnosis comes down to individual preference. Some like it. It can provide a framework to work from. Others aren't such a fan. They don't like labels and don't find them useful.

## Short-term burnout recovery

Recovering from burnout can take time, trial, and error. If we try to rush and try to do too much too quickly, then it can sometimes make it worse.

In the short term, burnout recovery is about resting and recovering our energy levels. This can often mean:

- Getting our sleep routines back in check.
- Eating a balanced diet – this doesn't mean that we have to go on a diet or lose weight. It's more about eating a range of foods at appropriate times and having proper meals rather than grabbing a coffee for breakfast and a chocolate bar for lunch.
- Taking some time out to do things that we enjoy.
- Reconnecting with family and friends.
- Having fun.
- Taking some time to be quiet and still – perhaps engaging in yoga, meditation, journaling, mindfulness, or another reflective activity.
- Noticing our alcohol consumption and getting it back under control if needed.
- Practising self-soothing.
- Assessing our self-care routines and see if we need to get back on top of anything we've let slide.

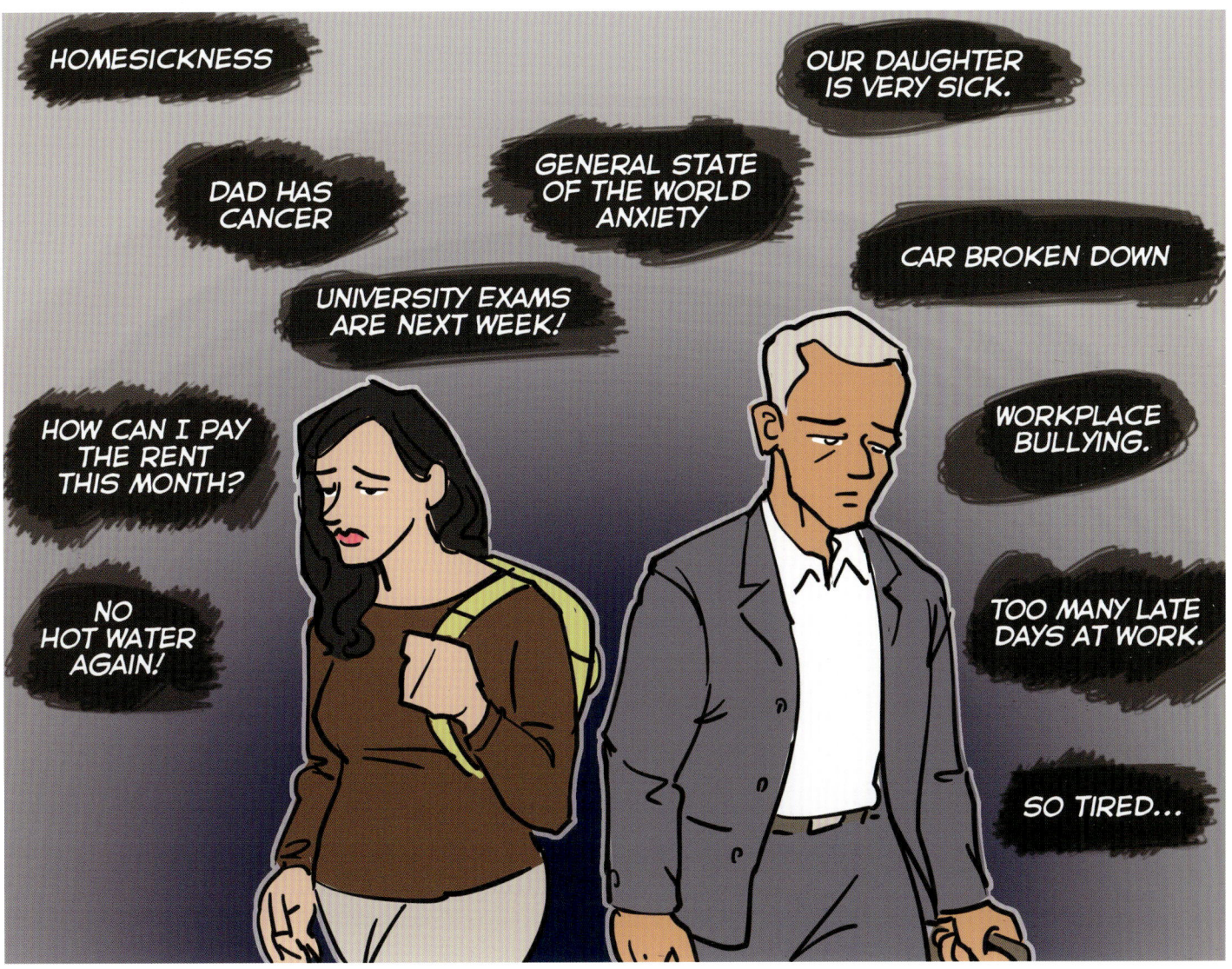

As we begin to feel better, we can start to look at those things we can do to prevent burnout going forward.

### Boundaries, priorities, and thank yous

As we recover from burnout, it's important to look at what caused it in the first place. Treating our symptoms is great, but unless we work out what's causing them, they'll just keep popping back up.

A stress log can be really helpful. To do this, we make a note each time we notice our anxiety or stress spike. Signs of an anxiety spike can include our heart rate speeding up, our breathing quickening, and we might suddenly feel very hot. Little stresses and annoyances can build and contribute to our overall stress levels. Making a note of them can allow us to do something about them.

Sorting out our wonky boundaries is important when preventing burnout. These could be work boundaries, people boundaries, or boundaries related to our own actions and behaviour. For example, one of our boundaries might be to leave work at work, but we might have started bringing bits and bobs home.

Reassessing different parts of our life can help us to view things from new perspectives and adjust our priorities accordingly. As part of this, we might need to delegate tasks, book some annual leave, have difficult conversations, and think about new boundaries or routines that we'd like to implement.

Sometimes, situations can spiral. We take on a bit more, ignore the odd lack of a 'thank you', do an extra hour here and there, and before we know it, we've become the 'yes' person. We end up working silly hours, have no downtime, and nobody seems to recognise our efforts. A 'thank you' can go a long way. If we feel unappreciated and taken for granted, then it might be important to talk to any relevant people about that. Conversations like this aren't easy but are important. During these conversations, it's also important that we stick to our new boundaries and priorities, reaffirming them as needed.

### Healthy habits

Preventing burnout isn't just about the situation that caused it, it also involves our wider life. The happier and healthier we are more generally, the more headspace we have to cope with ups and downs.

These healthy habits could include having a sensible bedtime, eating a balanced diet, making sure we have time off, having fun, connecting with nature, picking up forgotten hobbies, and communicating with those around us. Anything that forms part of our general self-care.

It's also useful to have a mental, written or physical toolkit of things that we can pull out during particularly difficult times. For example, if we've got a project deadline approaching then perhaps we need to ensure that for the two weeks beforehand, we step back from responsibilities elsewhere. Or if we come home having had a horrible day, then we might have a self-soothe box that we can dip into.

### We're not alone

It's important to remember, that whatever our situation, we're not alone. We're not the first person to feel this way. There are always things that we can do to try and improve our situation. When we feel our stress levels building, it's good to try and dial-up our self-care, reach out to those around us and try to prevent the stress from spiralling.

*18 March 2021*

The above information is reprinted with kind permission from *Blurt*
© 2022 The Blurt Foundation CIC

www.blurtitout.org

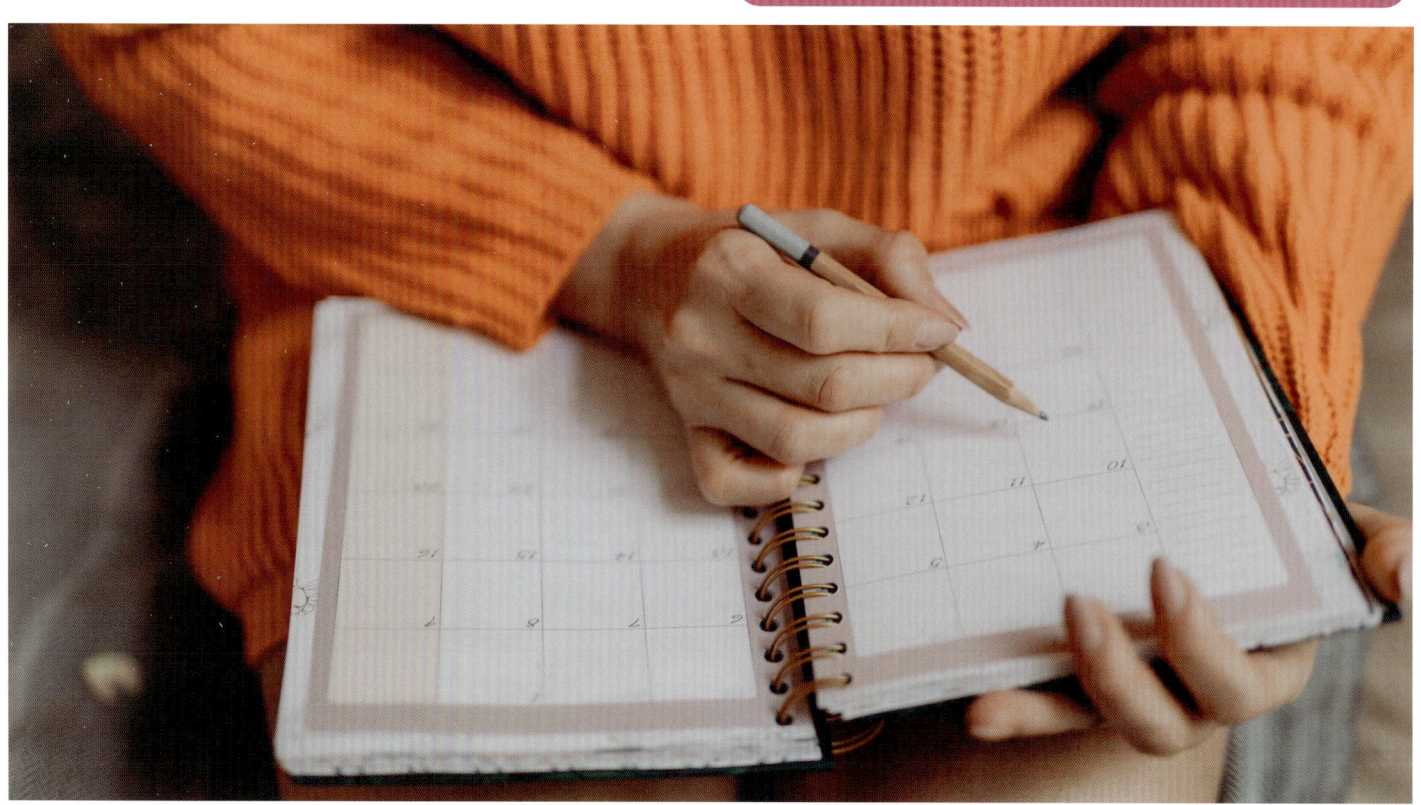

# Depression and anxiety rose sharply over Christmas in the UK

Levels of depression and anxiety rose sharply over December in the UK, especially among young adults, reaching similar levels to lockdown at the start of 2021, according to new findings from the Covid-19 Social Study led by UCL researchers.

Levels of depression and anxiety rose sharply over December in the UK, especially among young adults, reaching similar levels to lockdown at the start of 2021, according to new findings from the Covid-19 Social Study led by UCL researchers.

The research also found that confidence in devolved governments' handling of Covid-19 fell in England and Wales over the same period (between the end of November and start of January), but remained steady in Scotland. In England, the level of confidence was close to the lowest level recorded during the pandemic back in October 2020.

The new findings are based on a survey of 31,151 people taken in the first week of January 2022 as part of the ongoing Covid-19 Social Study, which has regularly surveyed more than 70,000 respondents since March 2020, tracking people's experiences of the pandemic. The study is funded by the Nuffield Foundation, UKRI and Wellcome.

The new survey also found a drop – compared to the last survey, conducted in the week of 22-28 November – in reported life satisfaction and happiness, with life satisfaction and happiness reaching their lowest levels since March 2021.

Lead author Dr Daisy Fancourt (UCL Institute of Epidemiology & Health Care) said: 'The findings reported here highlight the ongoing adverse effects of the pandemic on mental health. Even though there were many fewer restrictions this Christmas compared with Christmas 2020, levels of anxiety and depression were on a par with the same time last year. Our findings suggest that it is not just the presence of social restrictions that affect mental health but also concerns and stressors relating to high levels of the virus and a high risk of infection.

'The decrease in confidence in government to handle the pandemic likely contributed to the stresses many people faced over this period.'

In terms of people's concerns about Covid-19, the survey showed that the proportion of people concerned about catching or becoming seriously ill from Covid-19 increased sharply over the Christmas period, with:

- 43% of respondents saying catching Covid-19 was a major concern
- 46% worried about becoming seriously ill from Covid-19
- 58% concerned about family or friends catching Covid-19
- 52% reporting that the possibility of developing long Covid was a major concern

Three in four (73%) people reported being concerned about non-Covid-19 NHS treatment being cancelled, postponed or otherwise adversely affected over the next three months. Sixty-four per cent of respondents also had a major worry about hospitals being overwhelmed. These fears were greatest amongst adults over the age of 30 compared to adults aged 18-29.

Meanwhile, 86% of respondents reported that their experiences and behaviours had been different over the Christmas period compared to typical Christmases, such as staying at home more, changing travel plans, meeting up with fewer people, shopping online rather than in-store, avoiding large gatherings, and making fewer plans. Younger adults (aged 18-29) reported the fewest differences to usual compared to older adults.

Compliance with guidelines to prevent the spread of Covid-19 slightly increased over the Christmas period, indicating that people tightened up their behaviours. This pattern was seen clearly in 30- to 59-year-olds and 60+ year-olds. However, only four in 10 (43%) people said they currently understood the rules fully or near fully and one in 10 (10%) said they did not understand them at all.

Cheryl Lloyd, Education Programme Head at the Nuffield Foundation, said: 'In addition to the increase in depression and anxiety over the Christmas period, it is worrying that the majority of people report not fully understanding the current 'rules' in place to prevent the spread of Covid-19. This demonstrates there is an important communication challenge to be addressed by the government, so that people understand these rules – which have been subject to changes in recent weeks – and can comply with them.'

Older adults were more likely over the Christmas period to maintain a safe distance when meeting (30% always for those aged 60+ vs 9% of those aged 18-29) as well as washing their hands, wearing face masks, increasing ventilation in indoor spaces and meeting outdoors, but adults under the age of 60 were more likely to take lateral flow tests and ask others to take them, the survey found.

*19 January 2022*

The above information is reprinted with kind permission from *University College London*
©2022 UCL

www.ucl.ac.uk

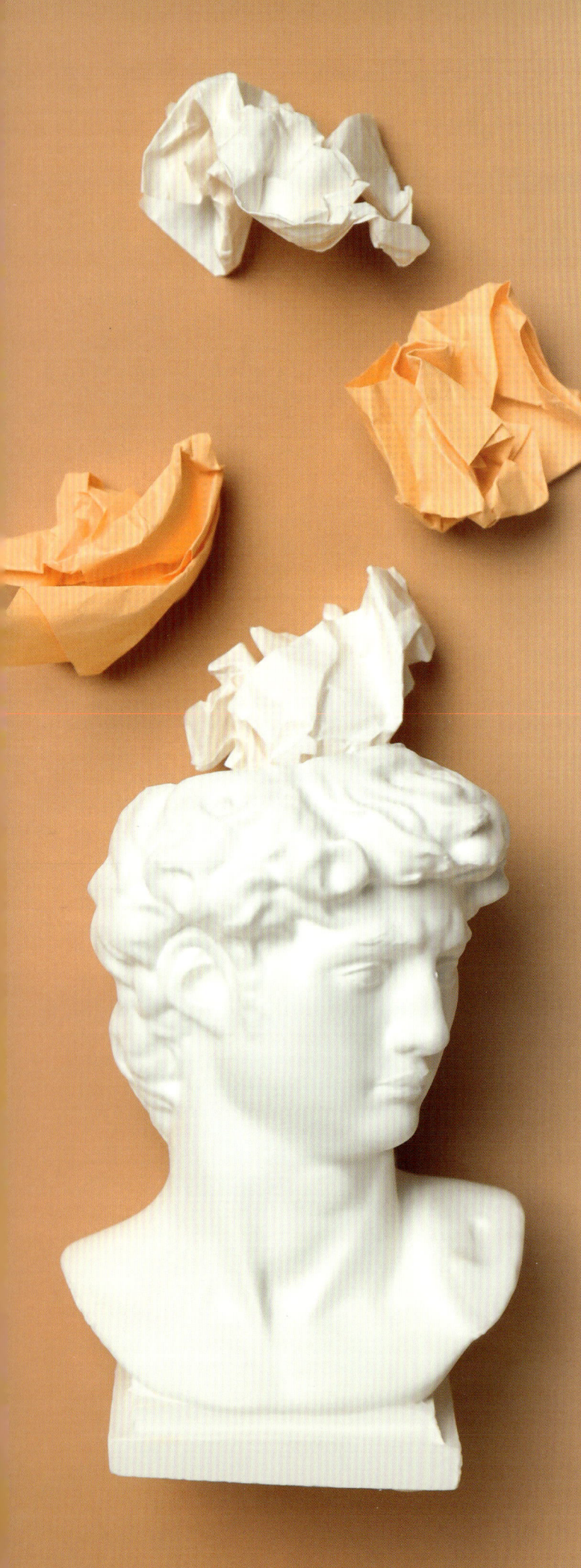

# People with depression can sometimes experience memory problems – here's why

An article from *The Conversation*.

By Cynthia Fu, Professor of Affective Neuroscience, University of East London

**THE CONVERSATION**

While we often associate depression with low mood, tiredness and feelings of hopelessness, less well known is that some people with depression may experience problems with their memory – such as feeling more forgetful than usual. Though memory problems aren't discussed as widely as other symptoms, we know that cognitive impairments are common in depression. In fact, up to three in five people with depression may experience them. It's thought that these memory problems are related to the changes in our brain's structure and function that happen because of depression.

Memory problems can occur when depression first begins, and can persist, even when other depressive symptoms have improved. Typically, it's our working memory that's affected. This is the short-term memory we use to actively remember things from moment to moment – and problems with it can make it difficult to concentrate or make decisions. In fact, many cognitive functions are often affected, such as response time, attention and planning, decision-making and reasoning. Depression also makes it difficult for our brain to switch between tasks and to inhibit what can be knee-jerk responses.

The severity of memory problems can vary from person to person. But some research shows cognitive impairments tend to be smaller in the first episode of depression, while worse memory problems have been seen with more severe depressive symptoms and repeated episodes of low mood. These effects on memory can even last when there are few or no symptoms of depression.

## Brain structure and function

Depression is linked to widespread changes in brain structure and function – including in the prefrontal cortex, hippocampus, and amygdala. These regions are all involved in cognition, executive function (such as planning, decision-making, and reasoning), and emotion processing.

These regions are interlinked via neural circuits, and they send and receive messages from each other, so problems in one region will impact on others. And, the neural circuits responsible for cognition and emotion processing overlap with those that control our stress response systems. So periods of high stress can also impair cognitive function and worsen mood.

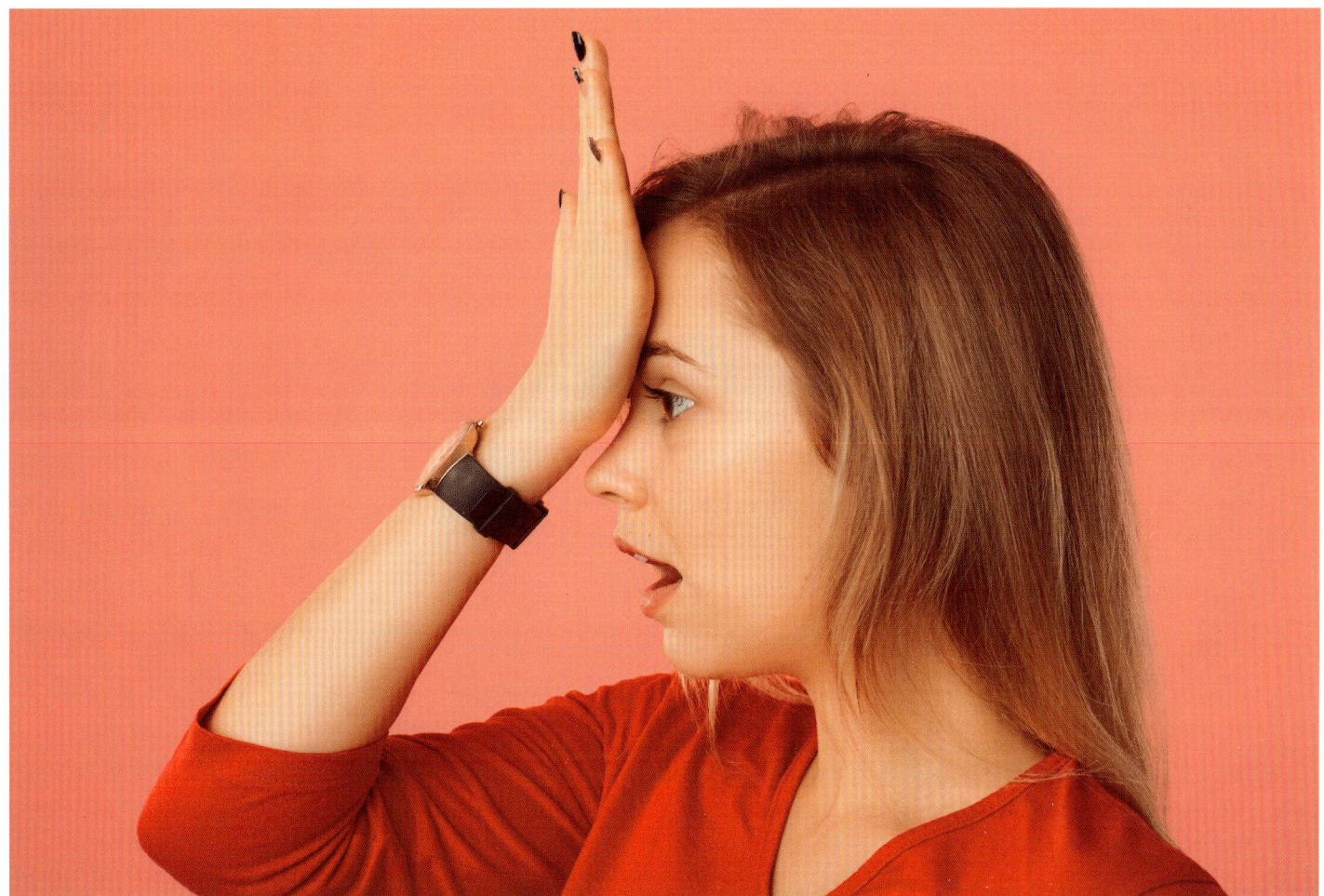

The changes in these brain regions seen in depression can have a big impact on how well our brain works during memory tasks. For example, people with depression often have a smaller hippocampus, and had increased activity extending from the prefrontal cortex during a working memory task in which they were asked to remember specific letters.

This meant the brains of people with depressiom had to work harder during the memory task by recruiting the help of additional brain regions to perform at the same level as participants who didn't have depression.

The circuits that connect cognition (including memory) and emotion use chemical messengers – such as serotonin, dopamine, noradrenaline and glutamate – which allow neurons in these brain regions to communicate with each other. Since brain messenger systems are continually interacting with each other, changes within them mean our neurons may be less able to communicate with each other. This may also affect how our memory works.

### Working memory

This isn't to say there aren't still many things a person struggling with depression can do to improve their memory.

For example, exercise is shown to benefit working memory, processing speed, and attention. It's thought that exercise releases brain messengers (including serotonin and dopamine) and increases activation in the brain's cortex. These both increase the growth of new neurons and brain plasticity (the brain's ability to change, adapt and grow). All of this is important for good memory.

Talking therapies also show increased activation in the prefrontal cortex, which could be linked with improved responsiveness and flexibility, both important aspects of cognition and mood. Cognitive training programs – such as cognitive exercises or games, usually done on a computer – can even improve working memory and attention.

In some cases, antidepressants can help to improve working memory. The most commonly prescribed antidepressants, selective serotonin reuptake inhibitors (SSRI) and serotonergic-noradrenergic reuptake inhibitors (SNRI), are also associated with improvements in planning, decision-making and reasoning – though these findings are mixed, and may not work as well for older people. Novel brain stimulation treatments, which affect how neurons can send signals, have also been associated with improvements to cognitive functions.

Memory problems can be a common symptom of depression and can have a serious impact on our day-to-day lives, including how well we perform at work and our relationships with other people. This is why it's important to consider memory problems alongside other core symptoms in depression – such as low mood – to improve treatment and prevent recurrence.

*9 February 2021*

The above information is reprinted with kind permission from The Conversation.
© 2010-2022, The Conversation Trust (UK) Limited

**www.theconversation.com**

# A changing brain: how depression can alter our brain structure

We've always known that mental illness and physical illness are intrinsically interlinked and inseparable. As more research is done into depression, researchers are discovering that it can alter our brain structure. It's hoped that research in this area could lead to better treatment and less stigma.

## Brain structure might sound like science fiction

The thought of depression changing our brain structure could feel scary or anxiety-provoking.

Though it might seem scary, these changes rarely occur in milder or shorter-term forms of depression. For those with Major Depressive Disorder (MDD), the good news is that with the right treatment some effects on the brain are reversible, and new treatments are being developed all the time.

The more we understand how depression interacts with our brain, the more we can learn about how it affects our functioning. This means that as well as investigating possible medical treatments, we can also look at non-medical interventions to help us manage life with any deficits we have.

Research on the brain is being done all the time and new discoveries are being made. Some of the discoveries around depression and the brain are very tentative, so we've covered those that are most understood and accepted.

## Bits of the brain

Before we look at brain structure, it can be helpful to have definitions for some parts of the brain

- Amygdala: The amygdala perches on top of our hippocampus, inside the temporal lobe. It's responsible for pleasure and fear, in charge of aggression, and helps to store memories of events and emotions.
- Frontal Lobe: The front section of our brain. It controls lots of things including problem-solving, inhibitions, expressing emotions, personality, concentration, mental flexibility, and organisation.
- Hippocampus: Our hippocampus sits at the bottom of our temporal lobe. It stores memories and regulates how much cortisol gets released.
- Hypothalamus: The hypothalamus lives in our temporal lobe, but sits in the top left of it. It creates and controls hormones, helps us to regulate our temperature, controls our appetite, tells us when we're thirsty, is in charge of our sleep cycles, is involved in sex drive and childbirth, and plays a part in our blood pressure and heart rate. It's very busy!
- Pre-Frontal Cortex: Our pre-frontal cortex lives at the front of our frontal lobe. It helps us out with lots of executive functions including focus, managing our emotions, impulse control, coordinating, and planning. It's also got a big part in our personality development.
- Temporal Lobe: This is a part of our brain that sits under our frontal lobe and on top of our brain stem. It holds our amygdala, hypothalamus, and hippocampus. It helps us with understanding language, organisation and sequencing, retrieving information, being aware of music, memory, hearing, learning, and our feelings.

## Key terms involved in brain structure

It's also helpful to have an understanding of some terms that relate to brain structure including:

- Brain-Derived Neurotrophic Factor (BDNF): For a simple protein, BDNF has a very long name! It's a protein that regulates the growth of our nerve cells.
- Cortisol: A hormone that's released when we're stressed. It's also involved in our parasympathetic nervous system.
- C-reactive protein (CRP): CRP is a protein that the liver makes. It hangs around in our blood and appears after injury, infection, or inflammation.
- Neurodegenerative: 'neuro' means nerve and 'degeneration' describes deterioration over time. Neurodegenerative describes the loss of nerve cells over time.
- Neuron: A neuron is another word for a nerve cell. It sends and receives nerve impulses.
- Neuroplasticity: Neuroplasticity describes how our brain changes as we age. It's about our brain responding to things we've learned and forming and reorganising different connections. Problems with it can cause changes in our pre-frontal cortex and hippocampus.
- Neurotransmitter: Neurotransmitters are chemicals that carry nerve impulses across a synapse (the gap between two nerve cells or a nerve cell and an organ).

## Brain shrinkage

When we have depression, parts of our brain can shrink.

Brain shrinkage is just as it sounds; parts of our brain reduce in size. The amount of shrinkage usually depends on how severe our depression is and how long we've lived with it.

When a section shrinks, the functions of that section 'shrink' too. This explains why some things we've previously done almost without thinking can become so difficult when we live with depression. Brain shrinkage can affect our hippocampus, thalamus, amygdala, frontal lobe, and prefrontal cortex.

Some shrinkage can be reversed with the right treatment. Studies have shown that people in remission from depression have bigger a hippocampus than those who aren't in remission, for example.

### Brain inflammation

C-reactive protein (CRP) is an indication of inflammation, infection, or injury. Those of us who live with depression could have up to 30% more CRP in our blood than those who don't.

Brain inflammation can cause our brain cells to die. This means that, counter-intuitively, inflammation can cause parts of our brain to shrink, changing our brain structure.

Inflammation can stop our neurotransmitters from working as well as they should do. This means that messages aren't passed through our body as effectively as they might be if we didn't have any inflammation. It also creates problems with neuroplasticity, so our brain isn't as able to change as we age. This can mean that we struggle to learn or adapt to any changes going on around us.

### Cortisol: a hormone with a big difference

One of the functions of our hippocampus is to regulate the amount of cortisol in our body. Cortisol is a hormone that's released when we're stressed. In the short-term, it's usually helpful. But when we live with long-term stress, for example when living with depression, our cortisol levels remain high which can start to cause problems.

Our hippocampus is full of a protein called 'brain-derived neurotrophic factor' (BDNF). It's really important for neuron growth and survival. High levels of cortisol can directly affect BDNF, stopping it from working properly.

High cortisol levels affect our neurons in other ways, too. It allows more calcium into our active neurons which damages them, causes the neurons in our hippocampus to shrink, and slows down the production of new neurons.

And that's not all it does. Cortisol also impacts our amygdala, causing it to become enlarged and more active. An enlarged, over-active amygdala then releases irregular amounts of hormones, causing more problems further down the line.

### Prefrontal cortex and brain structure

Our pre-frontal cortex is vital for a variety of functions including emotion regulation, language processing, impulse control, judgement, planning, and decision making. Teenagers are often stereotyped as making seemingly bizarre decisions, lacking impulse control and struggling to manage their emotions. One of the reasons for this is because a teenager's prefrontal cortex is still developing so skills associated with our pre-frontal cortex are often still developing, too.

When too much cortisol is released, it causes our prefrontal cortex to shrink. Having a smaller prefrontal cortex can mean that we struggle to make decisions, have poor impulse control, and find it hard to regulate our emotions, among other things.

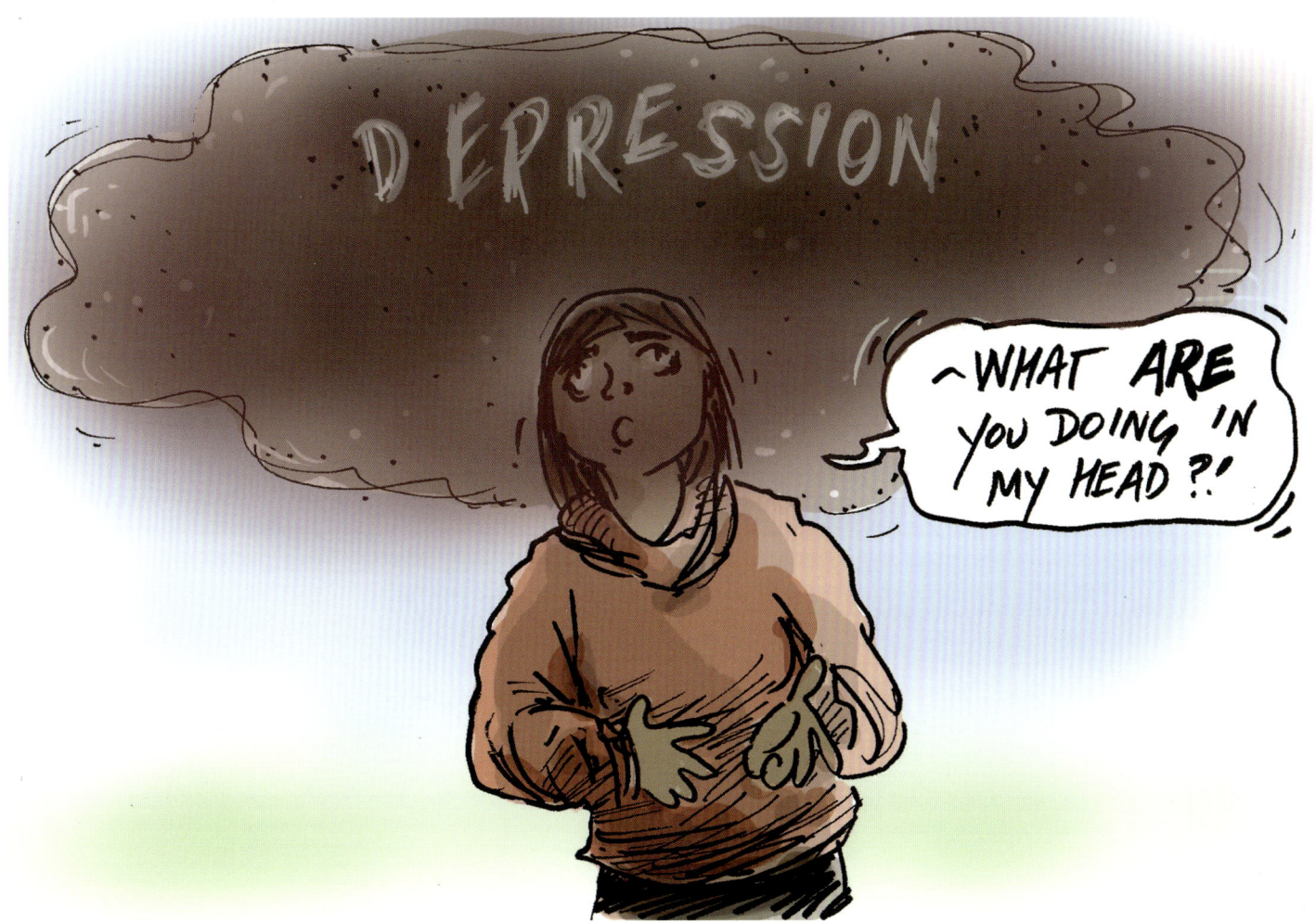

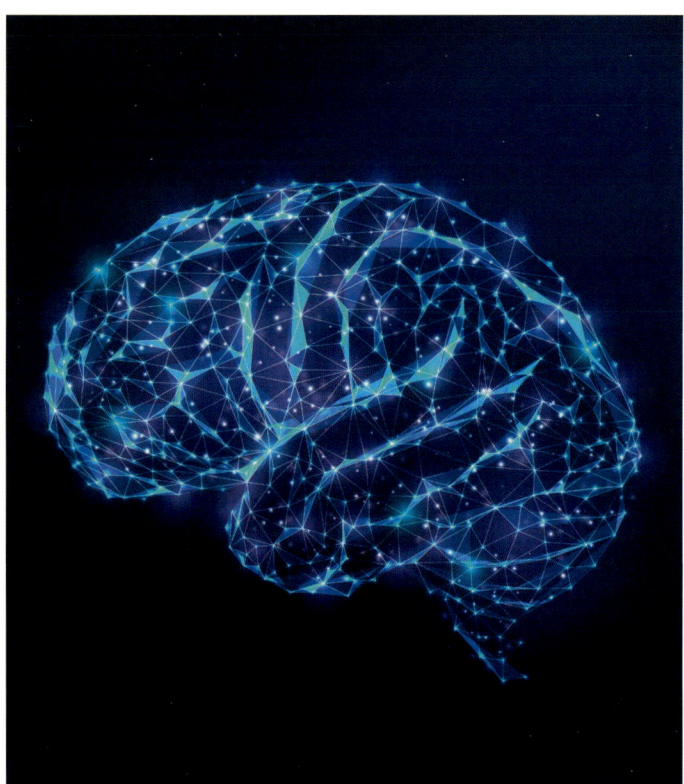

## What does all of this mean?

Any structural brain changes can take a minimum of eight months to appear so are far more common in those with persistent depression. We can't see inside our brain (unless we're in a scanner) so we can't visibly see any structural changes. However, we are likely to notice the effects of these changes.

Each part of our brain has a different function. Our frontal lobe takes care of things like problem-solving, inhibitions, judgements, planning, learning, expressing emotions and concentration. The prefrontal cortex, specifically, takes care of language processing, decision making, impulse control, planning, and emotional regulation. Feelings of pleasure and fear are controlled by our amygdala. It's also involved in the regulation of things like our sleep patterns. Our hippocampus affects our memory, including our verbal memory.

With a changing brain structure affecting all of these things and more, it's no wonder that depression can cause so many problems with functioning and mood.

## The effects of medical treatment

Medication can help to balance our hormones and other chemicals in our brain. This could reverse some of the structural changes that occur in our brain when we have depression, improving some of our symptoms. Antidepressants can also help to get our neural growth and activity going again.

As well as medication, there are some medical procedures which can help to reduce symptoms of major depression by targeting our brain. For example, Electroconvulsive therapy (ECT) and transcranial magnetic stimulation (TMS) can boost communication between our nerve cells and help to regulate our mood.

## Other things that can help

There are things that we can do both to prevent some of these changes and to reverse or improve them once they occur.

Stress can exacerbate depression and have a big impact on our cortisol levels. We know that this can alter our brain structure. Unfortunately, reducing our stress levels isn't usually as simple as just deciding not to be stressed. It often takes conscious effort over time. We have to notice the things that elevate our stress levels and then work to do something about them one at a time.

Some life changes can alter our brain structure. Eating a balanced diet and staying active (within reason) stimulate our brain cells and strengthen the communication between them. Sleeping gives our brain cells the chance to grow and repair. Alcohol and drugs can destroy our brain cells, so avoiding them can be a good idea.

Talking therapies, specifically psychotherapy, could alter the brain structure, too. Researchers think that psychotherapy can help to strengthen our prefrontal cortex, helping us with decision-making, memory-formation, and emotion-regulation.

## Increasing our understanding of brain structure

All of these brain changes can be a lot to take in, especially when they involve some long, scientific, words that are totally new to us. It can sound really scary and overwhelming.

The good news is that the more we understand what's going on, the more we can do about it. An increased understanding of the specific chains of events and mechanisms involved in depression allows researchers to create more specific treatments with better outcomes.

Researchers are also hopeful that learning about how depression can alter our brain structure will help to reduce the amount of stigma that some people hold when it comes to depression because they'll be able to see how it physically affects our body.

A lot of hope can be placed in the knowledge that science is advancing all of the time.

*1 October 2020*

The above information is reprinted with kind permission from *Blurt*
© 2022 The Blurt Foundation CIC

www.blurtitout.org

# Night owls more likely to be depressed because they have to work against their natural body clock, says study

By Ellen Scott

When you're more of a night owl than an early lark, you have a couple of options.

Either you find a job that has flexible enough hours to work around your ideal schedule, or you push through, do the traditional 9 to 5, and wander around in a near-constant state of bleary-eyed exhaustion.

Our society is set up to match the natural sleep and wakefulness flows of early risers, who are at their most awake and productive during the daytime.

So when you're naturally disposed to stay up late and struggle to wake up before 7am, things are tough.

And this might cause depression, suggests new research.

People whose sleep pattern goes against their natural body clock – meaning they are forced to go to bed and wake up earlier or later than they'd like – are more likely to have depression and lower levels of wellbeing, according to the study.

Researchers at the University of Exeter looked at previous research, which covered the genes linked to being an early riser or a night owl.

They then examined whether these genes were linked with certain health conditions, including depression.

As well as looking at genetic information, researchers also asked participants to complete a questionnaire on whether they were a morning person or better suited to the evenings.

Plus, they developed a measure of 'social jetlag' – the differences in sleep pattern between days people are working and days they're not.

They measured this in more than 85,000 UK Biobank participants for whom sleep data was available, via wrist-worn activity monitors.

Their findings add weight to suggestions that workplaces need to offer more flexible office hours to allow people to work with their body clock rather than against it. The researchers found that people who were more misaligned from their natural body clock were more likely to report depression and anxiety, and have lower wellbeing overall.

Lead author Jessica O'Loughlin said: 'We found that people who were misaligned from their natural body clock were more likely to report depression, anxiety and have lower wellbeing.

'We also found the most robust evidence yet that being a morning person is protective of depression and improves wellbeing.

'We think this could be explained by the fact that the demands of society mean night owls are more likely to defy their natural body clocks, by having to wake up early for work.'

Senior author Dr Jessica Tyrrell added: 'The Covid-19 pandemic has introduced a new flexibility in working patterns for many people.

'Our research indicates that aligning working schedules to an individual's natural body clock may improve mental health and wellbeing in night owls.'

*8 June 2021*

The above information is reprinted with kind permission from *Metro* & DMG Media Licensing.
© 2021 Associated Newspapers Limited

www.metro.co.uk

# Does depression exist?

Nobody understands why therapy works.

By Stuart Ritchie

It's not as strange a question as it might sound. Does depression exist? I don't mean to imply that those with depression should just 'pull themselves together': of course depression symptoms exist (and are sometimes life-ruining). And of course those symptoms often overlap with each other, which certainly implies that there's a common cause. But is there a thing we can point to in someone's brain – or some identifiable part of their psychology – that's called 'depression'?

In their understandable desire to get on with trials that might help people who are suffering, many researchers have sidestepped the question of what depression actually is. Instead, they've simply agreed on a definition and stuck to it. The Beck Depression Inventory is a questionnaire routinely used to diagnose and define depression: if you've ever spoken to your GP about feeling low, you might have come across it. It's named after Aaron Beck, one of the most important figures in the history of psychiatry (who died aged 100 on November 1st this year). He came up with 21 questions that cover guilt, feelings of failure, weight loss, insomnia, and suicidal thoughts, among other common depressive complaints.

The problem is that the medical profession, and psychiatry researchers, might be relying a little too much on that list of symptoms. Indeed, in an odd, unintentional, circular move, they might have actually turned lists of symptoms into the very definition of depression. An essay by the eminent psychiatrist Kenneth Kendler argues that this is a fundamental mistake: the number of boxes a patient ticks on the list of symptoms that get you a diagnosis isn't the same as 'depression' (nor is their Beck Depression Inventory score) – even if psychiatrists and researchers often act like it is. The Inventory is very often used as the criterion for improvement in studies of treatment: if you achieve a 50% drop in symptoms as measured on his questionnaire, you count as having been positively affected by the treatment. But these criteria are a decent index of many of the common symptoms – not all of them. We know anxiety commonly comes alongside depression, Kendler notes, but it's not on the standard diagnostic list. If we confuse the disease itself with a useful-but-limited list of its manifestations, we'll find it harder to truly understand patients' experiences.

Some researchers have gone a step further: should we stop using the concept of 'depression' entirely? One study of thousands of depression patients found over 1,000 unique combinations of symptoms that all still count as 'depression'. Maybe it's time, argue some, to focus on understanding subtypes, or even just specific symptoms, rather than the monolithic entity of 'depression' itself.

In some senses – and perhaps ironically – this accords with Beck's philosophy: he was known for being sceptical of focusing on the ultimate, root causes of mental illness. Which brings us to the other major contribution for which he is remembered: Cognitive Behavioural Therapy. Beginning in the 1960s, Beck reacted against the most popular form of therapy at the time, which was based on Freud's psychoanalytic theories of the mind. Beck – who himself was originally trained to administer psychoanalytic therapy

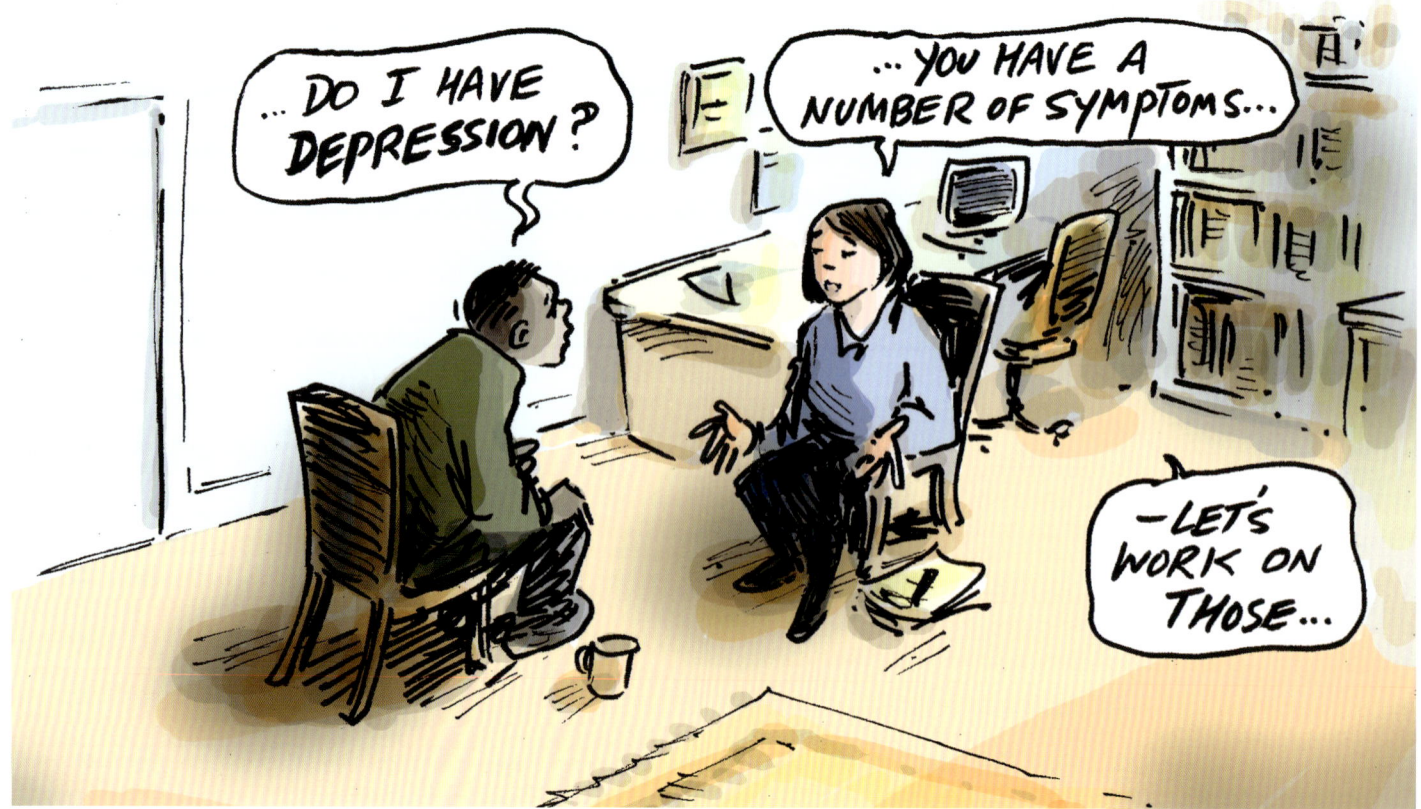

– began to doubt that depression symptoms were always caused by childhood traumas and unconscious repression. Some of the Freudian theories were rather far-fetched – as Tony Soprano says to his psychoanalytic therapist, after she suggests for the umpteenth time that he might be harbouring some Oedipal desires: 'I don't wanna fuck my mother! I don't give a shit what you say – you're never gonna convince me!'

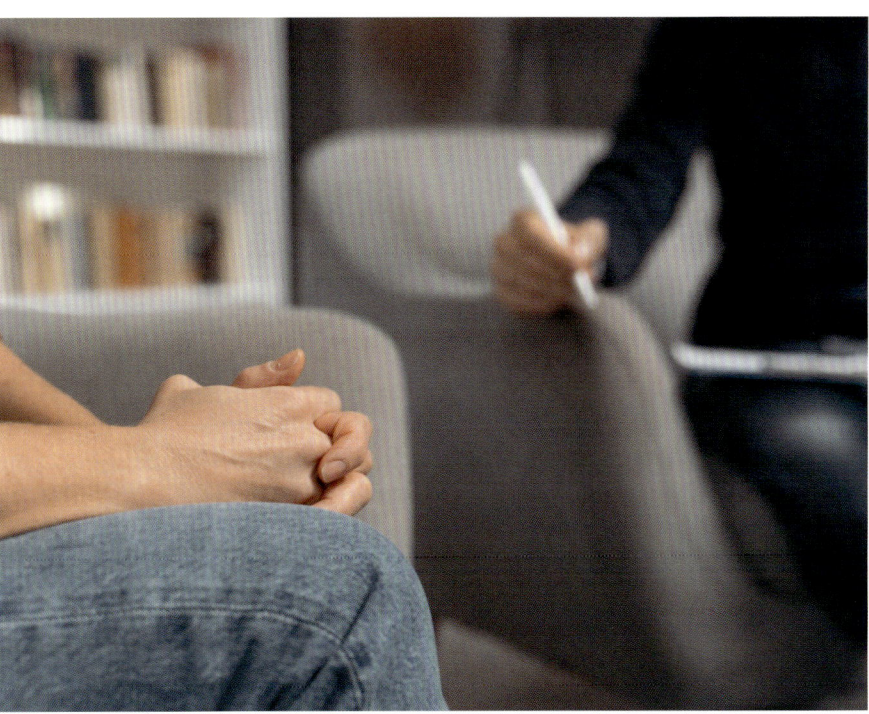

Instead, Beck suggested a much more proximal reason for the disorder: depression patients (and those with other disorders) are suffering from 'thought distortions'. For example, they might catastrophise, blowing minor unfortunate occurrences in life out of all proportion. They might overgeneralise, thinking that a fallout with one friend means that they're hated by everyone they know. As well as focusing his Depression Inventory on these kinds of thought patterns, Beck argued that therapy should target them and train patients out of them, rather than looking for some underlying explanation for all their symptoms.

Beck won the argument: although psychodynamic therapy still exists, CBT has now become the most popular – and by far the most studied – type of psychotherapy. New guidelines, announced this week, give patients the option of group CBT as the first line of treatment for mild depression; but even before then, it was extremely widely used. Its application goes well beyond depression: the language of CBT, with all its ideas about catastrophising and perfectionism and self-blame, is now, as Scott Alexander has memorably argued, 'in the water supply'. But 'popular' and 'culturally influential' doesn't necessarily mean 'good'. What do the studies say about whether it works?

Despite the sheer volume of research, the evidence is actually quite poor. The meta-analyses (reviews of all the studies that have looked at a particular question) do conclude that CBT works compared to doing nothing (a common control group, to which the therapy is compared, is made up of people who are on a waiting list for treatment). But it's worth remembering that positive studies are more likely to be published than ones concluding that the experiment in question doesn't work. And the overall literature on psychotherapy does show signs of this kind of bias.

So, even if the studies are right that CBT is beneficial (and in my view they most likely are), the extent of the benefit might be somewhat exaggerated. Those meta-analyses compare CBT to other common forms of psychotherapy, including the psychoanalytic kind (these days usually called 'psychodynamic' therapy). The general picture is this: the effects of CBT are essentially the same as any other kind of psychotherapy. They all reduce depression symptoms, and they all still seem to work up to a year later (this particular kind of meta-analysis has to assume all the trials are comparable, though – and that's often quite a big assumption).

It's a very similar story for drugs: the meta-analyses show that essentially all forms of antidepressant work better than placebo. But these effects are likely a bit overblown by all the dodgy practices in the scientific literature. And the evidence for one antidepressant being substantially better than another is, to use the kind of language one often sees in the review studies, 'limited' (which means researchers only have the vaguest clue).

Although this is good news in one sense, it's worrying (even depressing) in another. There is evidently a gaping hole in our evidence base on treating depression. If essentially all the major therapy types work to the same degree, despite being based on entirely different – often opposing – principles, it's pretty difficult to pin down exactly why they work. What exactly are the therapists doing in their sessions that makes the treatment effective? Can we really say that Beck was correct about CBT being the best treatment if other forms of therapy, which take an entirely different approach, can do the same job?

Maybe it doesn't matter whether therapists stick to Beck's plausible cognitive theories or Freud's absurd psychosexual ones. Maybe just having a regular interaction with a smart, sympathetic, well-organised person who focuses on your problems is what helps. That wouldn't explain, though, why the analyses showed that some forms of self-directed therapy can also make a difference. Either way, all this raises the question: how can we make our therapies better if we don't know the active ingredients? But then, how can we establish the active ingredients if we don't even know what we're treating?

**You can call Samaritans for free on 116 123, email them at jo@samaritans.org, or visit www.samaritans.org to find your nearest branch.**

*25 November 2021*

The above information is reprinted with kind permission from *UnHerd*.
©2022 UnHerd

**www.unherd.com**

# 'Overlooked and underfunded': experts call for global action to deal with depression

According to *The Lancet* and World Psychiatric Association Commission, the world is currently failing to tackle the persistent and increasingly severe global crisis of depression. Experts at the organisations have outlined an ambitious set of recommendations to tackle global inequities in diagnosis, treatment, and prevention, including prioritising an innovative staged approach to care and early intervention.

By Ed Brown

Globally, the World Health Organization estimates that 5% of adults worldwide suffer from depression each year. Nevertheless, it remains a neglected health crisis, which is frequently first experienced from the onset of adolescence.

Despite long-established research demonstrating that there is much that policymakers can be doing to prevent depression and aid recovery even in a resource-limited setting, in high-income countries, around half of the people suffering from depression are not diagnosed or treated. In contrast, this rises to 80-90% in middle-income countries.

The Covid-19 pandemic has created additional challenges, notably social isolation, bereavement, uncertainty, economic insecurity, and limited access to healthcare, which are all serious factors taking a severe toll on the mental health of millions worldwide.

Against this backdrop, *The Lancet* and World Psychiatric Association Commission's *Time for united action on depression* document calls for a concerted and collaborative effort by governments, healthcare providers, researchers, people living with depression, and their families to improve care and prevention efforts radically. The document has been written by 25 experts from 11 countries spanning disciplines from neuroscience to global health and has been advised by people with experience of depression.

## Childhood prevention and early intervention in adulthood

Commission Chair Professor Helen Herrman, National Centre for Excellence in Youth Mental Health, The University of Melbourne, Australia, described depression as a 'global health crisis' that requires a response on 'multiple levels'. By this, Prof Herrman and the Committee stressed that there needs to be a whole-of-society strategy to reduce exposure to both adverse experiences in childhood (such as by neglect and trauma) and across the lifespan to decrease the prevalence of depression through targeted intervention.

Dr Lakshmi Vijayakumar, Suicide Prevention Centre and Voluntary Health Services, Chennai, India, explained: 'Prevention is the most neglected aspect of depression. This [is] in part because most interventions are outside of the health sector.'

'In the face of the lifelong effects of adolescent depression, from difficulty in school and future relationships to risk of substance abuse, self-harm, and suicide, investing in depression prevention is excellent value for money.

It is crucial that we put into practice evidence-based interventions that support parenting, reduce violence in the family, and bullying at school, as well promoting mental health at work and addressing loneliness in older adults.'

## A more reflective, personalised, staged approach to care

The Commissioners recommend that the current system of classifying people with symptoms of depression into the categories of either clinical depression or not is abandoned. They argued that depression is far too complex a condition, with a wide range of symptoms, severity levels, and duration to be considered so simplistically.

Alternatively, experts at the Commission support the use of a personalised, staged approach to depression care, which recognises the chronology and intensity of symptoms tailored to an individual's symptoms.

Professor Vikram Patel, Commission Co-Chair, Harvard Medical School, USA, said:

'No two individuals share the exact life story and constitution, which ultimately leads to a unique experience of depression and different needs for help, support, and treatment. Similar to cancer care, the staged approach looks at depression along a continuum–from wellness to temporary distress, to an actual depressive disorder–and provides a framework for recommending proportional interventions from the earliest point in the illness.'

Furthermore, the Commission proposes adopting collaborative care strategies to scale up evidence-based intervention in routine care. In addition to combating the acute shortage of skilled providers and financial barriers to care, using locally recruited, low-cost non-mental health specialists, such as community health workers.

Although ultimately the team of experts concluded that far more significant investment globally is needed to ensure that everyone receives the care they need, where and when they need it.

*24 February 2022*

The above information is reproduced with kind permission of Pavilion Publishing and Media
© 2022 www.mentalhealthtoday.co.uk

www.mentalhealthtoday.co.uk

# Coping & Therapies

## In research studies and in real life, placebos have a powerful healing effect on the body and mind

An article from *The Conversation*.

By Elissa H. Patterson, Clinical Assistant Professor of Psychiatry and Neurology, University of Michigan & Hans Schroder, Clinical Assistant Professor of Psychiatry, University of Michigan

Did you ever feel your own shoulders relax when you saw a friend receive a shoulder massage? For those of you who said 'yes,' congratulations, your brain is using its power to create a 'placebo effect.' For those who said 'no,' you're not alone, but thankfully, the brain is trainable.

Since the 1800s, the word placebo has been used to refer to a fake treatment, meaning one that does not contain any active, physical substance. You may have heard of placebos referred to as 'sugar pills.'

Today, placebos play a crucial role in medical studies in which some participants are given the treatment containing the active ingredients of the medicine, and others are given a placebo. These types of studies help tell researchers which medicines are effective, and how effective they are. Surprisingly, however, in some areas of medicine, placebos themselves provide patients with clinical improvement.

As two psychologists interested in how psychological factors affect physical conditions and beliefs about mental health, we help our patients heal from various threats to well-being. Could the placebo effect tell us something new about the power of our minds and how our bodies heal?

### *Real-life placebo effects*

Today, scientists define these so-called placebo effects as the positive outcomes that cannot be scientifically explained by the physical effects of the treatment. Research suggests that the placebo effect is caused by positive expectations, the provider-patient relationship and the rituals around receiving medical care.

Depression, pain, fatigue, allergies, irritable bowel syndrome, Parkinson's disease and even osteoarthritis of the knee are just a few of the conditions that respond positively to placebos.

Despite their effectiveness, there is stigma and debate about using placebos in U.S. medicine. And in routine medical practice, they are rarely used on purpose. But based on new understanding of how non-pharmacological aspects of care work, safety and patient preferences, some experts have begun recommending increasing the use of placebos in medicine.

The U.S. Food and Drug Administration, the organization that regulates which medicines are allowed to go to the consumer market, requires that all new medicines be tested in randomized controlled trials that show they are better than placebo treatments. This is an important part of ensuring the public has access to high-quality medications.

But studies have shown that the placebo effect is so strong that many drugs don't provide more relief than placebo treatments. In those instances, drug developers and researchers sometimes see placebo effects as a nuisance that masks the treatment benefits of the manufactured drug. That sets up an incentive for drug manufacturers to try to do away with placebos so that drugs pass the FDA tests.

Placebos are such a problem for the enterprise of drug development that a company has developed a coaching script to discourage patients who received placebos from reporting benefits.

## Treating depression

Prior to the COVID-19 pandemic, about 1 in 12 U.S. adults had a diagnosis of depression. During the pandemic, those numbers rose to 1 in 3 adults. That sharp rise helps explain why US$26.25 billion worth of antidepressant medications were used across the globe in 2020.

But according to psychologist and placebo expert Irving Kirsch, who has studied placebo effects for decades, a large part of what makes antidepressants helpful in alleviating depression is the placebo effect – in other words, the belief that the medication will be beneficial.

Depression is not the only condition for which medical treatments are actually functioning at the level of placebo. Many well-meaning clinicians offer treatments that appear to work based on the fact that patients get better. But a recent study reported that only 1 in 10 medical treatments sampled met the standards of what is considered by some to be the gold standard of high quality evidence, according to a grading system by an international nonprofit organization. This means that many patients improve even though the treatments they receive have not actually been proved to be better than the placebo.

## How does a placebo work?

The power of the placebo comes down to the power of the mind and a person's skill at harnessing it. If a patient gets a tension headache and their trusted doctor gives them a medicine that they feel confident will treat it, the relief they expect is likely to decrease their stress. And since stress is a trigger for tension headaches, the magic of the placebo response is not so mysterious anymore.

Now let's say that the doctor gives the patient an expensive brand-name pill to take multiple times per day. Studies have shown that it is even more likely to make them feel better because all of those elements subtly convey the message that they must be good treatments.

Part of the beauty of placebos is that they activate existing systems of healing within the mind and body. Elements of the body once thought to be outside of an individual's control are now known to be modifiable. A legendary example of this is Tibetan monks who meditate to generate enough body heat to dry wet sheets in 40-degree Fahrenheit temperatures.

A field called Mind Body Medicine developed from the work of cardiologist Herbert Benson, who observed those monks and other experts mastering control over automatic processes of the body. It's well understood in the medical field that many diseases are made worse by the automatic changes that occur in the body under stress. If a placebo interaction reduces stress, it can reduce certain symptoms in a scientifically explainable way.

Placebos also work by creating expectations and conditioned responses. Most people are familiar with Pavlovian conditioning. A bell is rung before giving dogs meat that makes them salivate. Eventually, the sound of the bell causes them to salivate even when they do not receive any meat. A recent study from Harvard Medical School successfully used the same conditioning principle to help patients use less opioid medication for pain following spine surgery.

Furthermore, multiple brain imaging studies demonstrate changes in the brain in response to successful placebo treatments for pain. This is excellent news, given the ongoing opioid epidemic and the need for effective pain management tools. There is even evidence that individuals who respond positively to placebos show increased activity in areas of the brain that release naturally occurring opioids.

And emerging research suggests that even when people know they are receiving a placebo, the inactive treatment still has effects on the brain and reported levels of improvement.

## Placebos are nontoxic and universally applicable

In addition to the ever-increasing body of evidence surrounding their effectiveness, placebos offer multiple benefits. They have no side effects. They are cheap. They are not addictive. They provide hope when there might not be a specific chemically active treatment available. They mobilize a person's own ability to heal through multiple pathways, including those studied in the field of psychoneuroimmunology. This is the study of relationships between the immune system, hormones and the nervous system.

By defining a placebo as the act of setting positive expectations and providing hope through psychosocial interactions, it becomes clear that placebos can enhance traditional medical treatments.

## Using placebos to help people in an ethical way

The placebo effect is recognized as being powerful enough that the American Medical Association considers it ethical to use placebos to enhance healing on their own or with standard medical treatments if the patient agrees to it.

Clinically, doctors use the principles of placebo in a more subtle way than it is used in research studies. A 2013 study from the U.K. found that 97% of physicians acknowledged in a survey having used some form of placebo during their career. This might be as simple as expressing a strong belief in the likelihood that a patient will feel better from whatever treatment the doctor prescribes, even if the treatment itself is not chemically powerful.

There is now even an international Society for Interdisciplinary Placebo Studies. They have written a consensus statement about the use of placebos in medicine and recommendations for how to talk with patients about it. In the past, patients who improved from a placebo effect might have felt embarrassed, as if their ailment were not real.

But with the medical field's growing acceptance and promotion of placebo effects, we can envision a time when patients and clinicians take pride in their skill at harnessing the placebo response.

*11 February 2022*

The above information is reprinted with kind permission from The Conversation.
© 2010-2022, The Conversation Trust (UK) Limited

www.theconversation.com

# Piecing life back together after a period of depression

Piecing life back together following a period of depression isn't always straightforward. There are lots of things to consider and think about. It's often something we have to work really hard at.

## The straightforward recovery myth

There is a myth that recovery is a smooth, straight line. That all we have to do is take medication, go to therapy, use the skills we've been taught, and then we'll be okay again.

Unfortunately, that's not the case. Recovery is usually a wibbly-wobbly line with the odd loop-the-loop. When piecing life back together, there are times when things improve, and times when things seem to be getting worse again. Over time we can learn to manage our depression and many people will reach a point of recovery, but it isn't usually a straightforward process.

## The 'returning to our previous life' myth

Another myth is recovery means returning to the life we had before becoming unwell, exactly as it was. Although this might be possible for some people, it's usually an unrealistic goal.

Depression is rough. It puts us through some really awful times, and sends our mind to places it's never been before. It also teaches us things and can alter our perspective. We might have changed. Parts of our life could have changed. We might have to get used to managing or adapting certain areas of our life to stay well.

We're not the only ones affected, either. Our depression often affects everyone around us, too. People may have seen us in ways that we hoped they never would.

None of this is to say that we can't create a meaningful, fulfilling life. We absolutely can. But it's unlikely to look identical to our life pre-illness.

## Making changes when piecing life back together

If we go straight back to the environment that we became unwell in, then it might not serve us very well.

Making some changes to our life can help us to stay well longer-term.

We don't need to give our entire life a makeover. But making tweaks here and there, building in a healthy routine, and thinking about what lifts us up and what drags us down can help us to stay well.

Additionally, we might feel as though we've changed as a person. The things that used to interest us might not anymore. We could have developed a passion for something totally new.

Change can be scary, but staying the same can be scary, too.

## Take it slowly

When piecing our life back together it's often tempting to try and return to our 'normal life' as quickly as possible. Unfortunately, this can actually be detrimental to our recovery.

Part of recovery is carefully testing various aspects of life to see how they affect us. For example, we might be a volunteer lifeguard in our spare time. Through slowly returning to it, we might discover that we were doing too many shifts and

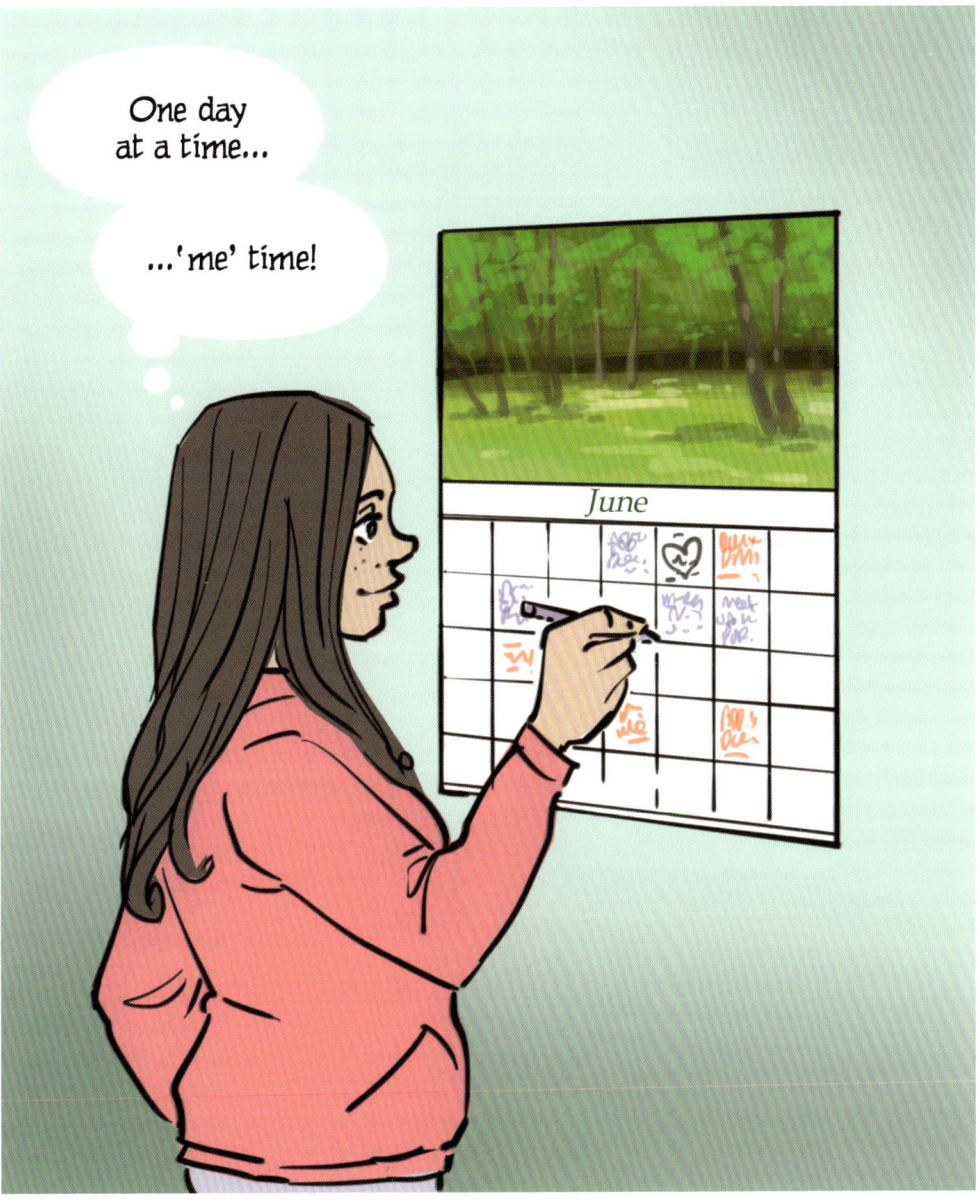

burning ourselves out; so we need to reduce them.

We might find that we cope well with some things and that they're really good for our mood. But there will also be parts of our life that we need to adjust.

If we return to lots of different things at once, then it can be much harder to tease out the things that are conducive to recovery, and those which are detrimental.

Doing things slowly can feel frustrating, but it enables us to make sustainable changes. It teaches us how to work out whether different activities help or hinder our mental health, allowing us to tweak them as necessary. This can be a useful, life-long skill.

### *Frustration*

Piecing our life back together can come with lots of frustration.

When we're really unwell, we often 'switch off' from life. We might not be interested in doing anything at all.

As we begin to recover our interest and motivation can begin to stir.

Unfortunately, even if we remember a certain task being 'easy', it might feel really difficult and take a huge amount of energy. Depression often clogs up our brain making it hard to think and affecting our executive functioning. Depending on how long we've been unwell, it might be ages since we did certain things, making it hard to remember everything involved.

It's so frustrating and can negatively impact our confidence. The thing is, if we've not done something in a really long time then, of course, we're going to find it difficult; anyone would! We need to try and be kind to ourselves. We will get there, it just takes time.

### *Confidence when piecing life back together*

Depression can take a sledgehammer to our confidence. It can make us feel useless and hopeless to the extent that we don't see any value in our life. As we start to piece life back together, low self-confidence often remains.

Re-building our self-confidence takes time, patience, self-kindness, and support.

### *The exhaustion of piecing life back together*

Piecing life back together is exhausting. We're doing things that we've not done in a long time. We might be moving more than we've done in a while, trying to make sense of lots of sensory information coming at us at once, and re-learning how to socialise and be around other people.

Depression is exhausting in itself. Recovery is exhausting, too. Put them both together and it's no wonder we're so tired.

If our body tells us that we need to rest, then we need to rest. We might be trying to do too much too fast. Some of our early warning signs could start to crop up. We might need to slow down and pull back a bit.

When we're about to tackle something new, we might want to create a ready-made 'safe spot' to come back to once we've done it. It could include blankets, headphones, and anything else we need to self-soothe.

### *Guilt and shame*

Guilt and shame can weigh heavily on our shoulders. When piecing life back together, we might remember things that we did or said when we weren't well. Other people might tell us about things we have no memory of.

We often feel guilty for how our depression affects those around us. We often don't want them to worry. They might have helped with practical things, like taking us

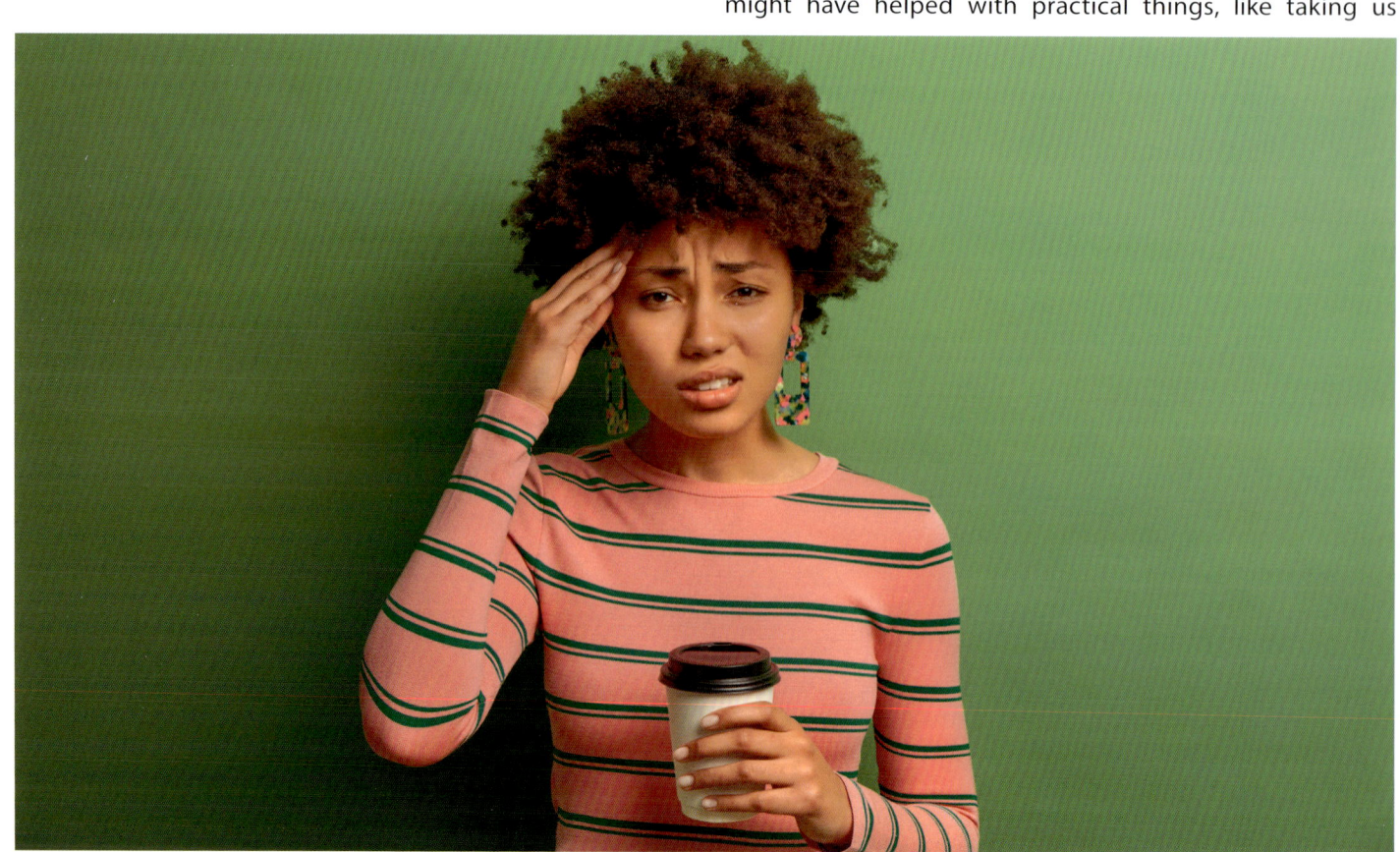

to appointments. We might have lost count of how often they've held us as we cried.

When people care about us, they're there for the good, the bad, and the ugly. We wouldn't shame our friends if they were feeling low and needed some support.

Depression can creep into all areas of our life. We might feel shame about our difficulties with personal hygiene, or guilty for asking our housemate to help us sort out or medication.

Depression is an illness. It's not an excuse, and should never be used as one, but it can be a reason for certain things. We didn't choose to have it and we can't just click our fingers and make it disappear (wouldn't that be nice?!). We have absolutely nothing to feel ashamed or guilty about.

### Things seem pointless

Some of us have experienced trauma pre-depression or during our depression. Our head could have taken us to some really dark places. We might have had some terrifying experiences. This can make conversations about footballers or soaps seem trivial, pointless, and vapid. It can be hard to join in.

We can care about both the state of the mental healthcare in our country and whether or not so-and-so marries whats-their-name on our favourite TV programme. We're not restricted to only caring about one thing at once. It's okay to be invested in things that might not seem to matter 'in the grand scheme of things'. We all need an escape sometimes.

### Leaving the house

Starting to leave the house after a period of illness can be tough. It could come with paralysing fear.

Our appearance might have changed; depression can alter our appetite, make it hard to clean our teeth, and generally make it tough to look after ourselves. This can negatively impact our confidence.

When we do begin to leave the house again, there's no rush. We can grade it, taking it step-by-step. 'Grading something', means to gradually increase the level of challenge, until we reach our goal. For example, if our goal is 'being able to go wherever whenever', then we might start by sitting on our front doorstep for five minutes, and build things up really slowly until we reach our overall goal.

### Learning to talk again

Depression can steal our voice.

Words can feel thick in our mouth. We might talk noticeably slowly because our brain is on go-slow mode. If we've become isolated, we might have gone days at a time without uttering a single word.

When we do start engaging with the world again, our voice might sound quite weird to us. It can be difficult to start getting our words out. We're out of practice.

The idea of 'practising to talk' might sound strange, but it can help us to improve the fluidity of our speech. We could chat with our pet, talk to ourselves, narrate what we're doing out loud, ring friends instead of messaging them, create short videos (such as Instagram stories), or try to talk to any delivery drivers or shop assistants we encounter.

Over time, talking should become second-nature to us again.

### Pushing people away

When unwell, we might push away everyone we've ever been close to. Irritability can make us snappy. We might have wanted to avoid hurting them so. We could have wanted to be left alone. This can understandably cause friction in relationships, but with open, honest conversations, we can often reignite these relationships.

If we've struggled to socialise for a while then we might feel 'out of the loop'. There's nothing helpful like a recap at the start of every chat and it can take us a while to catch up again. To begin with, it can feel more isolating than ever before. In time we'll get back to being 'in the loop' again. It can just take time.

### Friends

Going through a tough patch shows us who our real friends are, something that's not always easy to cope with.

When piecing life back together, people who haven't spoken to us since we became unwell might reappear. Of course, they might have had things going on in their own life that have coincided with our illness. But if they just decided that they couldn't cope with our depression then it might be time to re-evaluate our friendship.

### Family

Seeing how our depression impacts our family can be tough. They might tell us about the sleepless nights they've spent worrying about us, or get frustrated at us for something.

Communication is often key. We've haven't been through this rough patch in total isolation. To stop everyone's emotions from bubbling over, it's important to keep communication lines open. This doesn't just mean talking, but listening too. It probably won't be easy, but it's usually easier and more straightforward than the alternative.

### Children

One of the most painful things about depression is how it can impact any children we're regularly in contact with.

We may have our own children, or, regularly helped out with friends, or family's child(ren) before we became unwell. As we start to piece our life back together, discussions around childcare might crop up.

Children can be amazing for our recovery. But they're also never-ending bundles of energy.

It's really important to be honest with ourselves. Children are a responsibility and we may well need help (especially if we're caring for them alone).

### Where work comes into piecing life back together

Our job can take some tweaking, flexing, and trial and error until it feels okay. We spend lots of time there, so we need to try and arrange it in a way that works for us.

If that's not possible, we might choose to leave our job, apply for something else, or to retire altogether. For those of us who do choose to return to work, we do have certain rights. Having an idea of them can be handy.

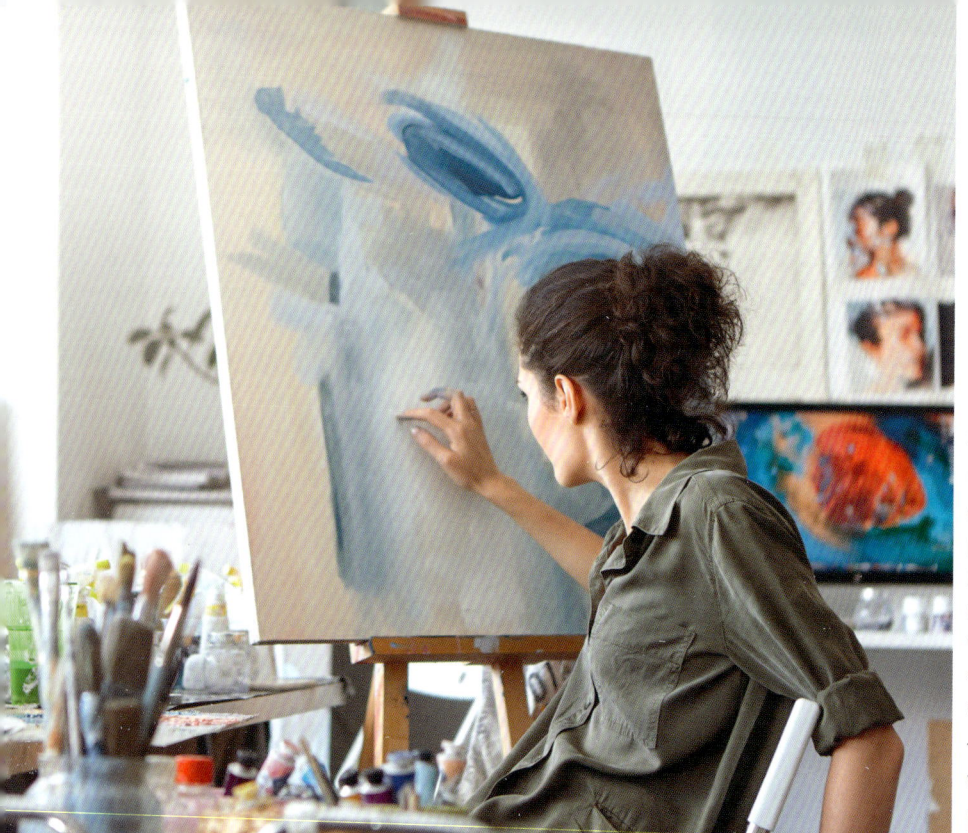

Adaptations we could ask for at work include things like having a graded return, doing some hours from home, flexitime, temporarily reducing our hours, steering clear of night shifts for a while, using headphones, and having more breaks.

For some of us, work is helpful, for others it's less so. But even if it's helpful, it can still be draining. We still need to try and balance it alongside everything else.

The Human Resources department (if we have one) might help us to put any adaptations we might need in place. They might recommend a referral to an Occupational Therapist. We might be able to directly refer ourselves to the Occupational Therapy department.

### Where education comes into piecing life back together

Unfortunately, education is sometimes less flexible than employment. If we've had some time off, there might be topics or modules that we've missed. We might miss certain lessons due to appointments, and need to catch up on them, too.

Staying on top of our school or university work while living with depression is hard. Trying to catch up any work we've missed on top of that adds another layer of stress and can become too much for us to handle.

It can be helpful to speak to a member of school or university staff about what our options are. There might be options that we haven't considered, such as spreading our work over a longer period, dropping subjects, or going to catch-up sessions.

### Hobbies

Hobbies often end up at the bottom of the priority pile. We might not view our hobbies as being 'as important' as our job, but they can be a big part of our recovery. They can help us to socialise, leave the house, engage with people, and find a sense of purpose and meaning.

### *Money, money, money*

When we're unwell, paying our bills can be tricky.

Firstly, if we've had to reduce our hours, take a pay cut, take sick leave, or we've been made redundant, then money can be tight.

Even if we can cover our bills, we might still procrastinate paying them. Depression can make it hard to think, especially when doing something that involves multiple steps, such as paying a bill.

Our paperwork pile can turn into a paperwork mountain. Bills add up (and so do the charges for not paying them on time). As we start to piece our life back together, we are often confronted with these piles, payments, and charges. This can be unbelievably stressful, come with a giant dollop of shame.

There's no shame in struggling with money. We don't need to struggle on alone. There are people we can talk to such as Citizens Advice, our bank, friends, and family. Places like MoneySupermarket.com have some fantastic advice, too. We aren't the first and won't be the last person to struggle with money and we deserve the help and support that we need to help us get back on track again.

### *Staying well after piecing life back together*

There will always be difficult things that crop up in life and our recovery is never going to be a smooth, straight line. But we can build certain things in our life to help us stay well.

This could include things like:

♦ Creating a balance of 'busy' and 'rest' time

♦ Thinking about our Early Warning Signs and sharing them with our loved ones

♦ Meal planning

♦ Setting a bedtime for ourselves

♦ Making a note of any skills that we've learned to manage our emotions so that we can use them when needed

♦ Creating a WRAP (Wellness Recovery Action Plan) and sharing it with loved ones

♦ Developing a solid self-care routine

♦ Setting rules or non-negotiables for ourselves (e.g. have a shower ever Sunday no matter how bad I feel)

We're all different so we'll all have different things that help us to stay well. The things that help might change as we go through life, too.

*27 August 2020*

The above information is reprinted with kind permission from *Blurt*
© 2022 The Blurt Foundation CIC

www.blurtitout.org

# NHS to give therapy for depression before medication under new guidelines

Draft guidance says 'menu of treatment options' including CBT and mindfulness should be offered in less severe cases.

*By Andrew Gregory*

Millions of people with mild depression in England should be offered therapy, exercise, mindfulness or meditation before antidepressants, according to the first new NHS guidelines in more than a decade.

Under draft guidance, the National Institute for Health and Care Excellence (NICE) recommends the 'menu of treatment options' be offered to patients by health professionals before medication is considered.

Currently, those with mild depression are offered antidepressants or a high-intensity psychological intervention, such as cognitive behavioural therapy (CBT). The shake-up forms part of the first new recommendations to identify, treat and manage depression in adults since 2009.

According to the Office for National Statistics (ONS), about one in six (17%) adults experienced some form of depression this summer. The rate is higher than before the pandemic, when 10% of adults experienced it. Younger adults and women are more likely to be affected, the ONS found.

A 2019 review showed 17% of the adult population in England (7.3 million people) had been prescribed antidepressants in the year 2017-18.

Dr Paul Chrisp, director of the centre for guidelines at NICE, said: 'The Covid-19 pandemic has shown us the impact depression has had on the nation's mental health. People with depression need these evidence-based guideline recommendations available to the NHS, without delay.'

Under the changes, those with 'less severe depression', which includes people with mild depression, should be involved in conversations with doctors about what would suit them best, but group cognitive behavioural therapy (CBT) could be offered as a first treatment. CBT 'focuses on how thoughts, beliefs, attitudes, feelings and behaviour interact, and teaches coping skills to deal with things in life differently'.

This could be followed by offers of seven other treatments including individual CBT, self help, group exercise or group mindfulness or meditation, before medication is discussed as an option.

Group exercise will typically involve three 60-minute sessions a week for 10 weeks, NICE said. Alternatively, patients could opt for group mindfulness or meditation, which NICE said usually consist of eight weekly two-hour sessions and focus on 'concentrating on the present, observing and sitting with thoughts and feelings and bodily sensations, and breathing exercises'.

The guideline adds: 'Do not routinely offer antidepressant medication as first-line treatment for less severe depression, unless that is the person's preference.'

A similar range of psychological interventions, along with the option of antidepressant medication, should be available to those choosing a first-line treatment for 'more severe depression'.

When considering treatment options, NICE said people should also be encouraged to discuss what may be contributing to their depression, and the patient's experience of any prior episodes of depression or treatments.

Nav Kapur, professor of psychiatry and population health at the University of Manchester and chair of the guideline committee, said: 'As a committee we have drawn up recommendations that we hope will have a real impact on people who are suffering from depression and their carers. In particular we've emphasised the role of patient choice – suggesting that practitioners should offer people a choice of evidence-based treatments and understanding that not every treatment will suit every person.'

The guidance recommends doctors discuss mental health waiting lists with patients. It also contains new recommendations for those stopping antidepressants.

People who are considering taking, or stopping, antidepressant medication should talk with their healthcare professional about the benefits and risks, NICE said. Doctors should explain that withdrawal may take weeks or months to complete successfully, that it is usually necessary to reduce the dose in stages over time, and that most people stop antidepressants successfully.

Figures from the NHS Business Services Authority show more than 20 million antidepressants were prescribed between October and December 2020 – a 6% increase compared with the same three months in 2019.

'There has been significant progress in science and medicine in the past 12 years,' said retired solicitor Catherine Ruane, a lay member on the guideline committee who acted as a carer to two family members with depression. 'This guideline emphasises a greater amount of patient choice and takes greater account of the things that really matter to the patients and their carers.'

*23 November 2021*

The above information is reprinted with kind permission from *The Guardian*.
© 2022 Guardian News and Media Limited

www.theguardian.com

# Ketamine therapy swiftly reduces depression and suicidal thoughts

Analysis of 83 research papers by academics at the University of Exeter showed that patients' symptoms were reduced in just one to four hours.

By Rod Minchin

The rave drug ketamine can quickly ease depression and soothe suicidal thoughts in the short term, research has revealed.

Analysis of 83 research papers showed that patients' symptoms were reduced in just one to four hours.

Some patients were relieved of suicidal thoughts for up to a week – though the average was three days.

The University of Exeter's review found that the strongest evidence emerged around the use of ketamine to treat both major depression and bipolar depression.

Lead author Merve Mollaahmetoglu said: 'Our research is the most comprehensive review of the growing body of evidence on the therapeutic effects of ketamine to date.

'Our findings suggest that ketamine may be useful in providing rapid relief from depression and suicidal thoughts, creating a window of opportunity for further therapeutic interventions to be effective.

'It's important to note that this review examined ketamine administration in carefully controlled clinical settings where any risks of ketamine can be safely managed.'

For other psychiatric disorders, including anxiety disorders, post-traumatic stress disorder and obsessive-compulsive disorder, there is early evidence to suggest the potential benefit of ketamine treatment.

'For individuals with substance use disorders, ketamine treatment led to short-term reductions in craving, consumption and withdrawal symptoms.

Senior author Professor Celia Morgan added: 'We're finding that ketamine may have promising benefits for conditions that are notoriously hard to treat in clinic.

'We now need bigger and better-designed trials to test these benefits.

'For example, due to ketamine's unique subjective effects, participants may be able to tell whether they have been given ketamine or a saline solution as the placebo, potentially creating an expectation about the effects of the drug.

'This effect may be better controlled by having active placebo-controlled trials, where the control group receives another drug with psychoactive properties.'

Questions remain unanswered in the research field, including the optimal dose, route of administration and number of doses of ketamine treatment.

There is also a need for further research on the added and interactive benefit of psychotherapy alongside ketamine treatment.

– The study, Ketamine for the treatment of mental health and substance use disorders: comprehensive systematic review, is published in the journal British Journal of Psychiatry Open.

*30 December 2021*

The above information is reprinted with kind permission from *The Independent*.
© independent.co.uk 2022

www.independent.co.uk

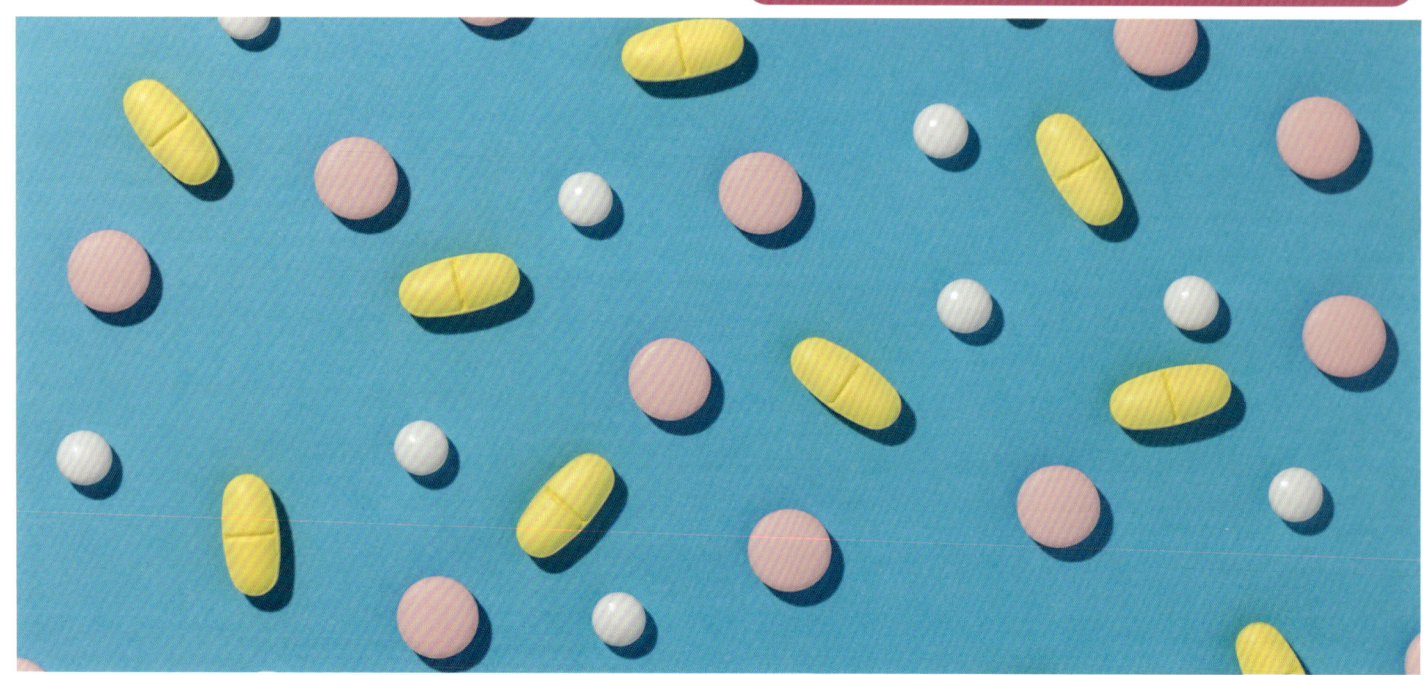

# A world without antidepressants: the new alternatives to prescription pills

Could the future of treating depression be ketamine infusions – or even a 'pacemaker for the brain'?

By David Cox

Five years ago, Mark Dunning was at his lowest ebb. After years of switching from one antidepressant medication to another without success, his mental health was worse than ever. 'I was suicidal,' he remembers. 'I'd been on various medications – sometimes they would work for a year or two and sometimes not at all. Those that did seem to work would abruptly stop with no warning at all and I literally couldn't see myself being alive anymore. I just felt hopeless and disinterested in everything I'd ever enjoyed.'

His experience is far from unique. One in five adults in the UK has symptoms of anxiety or depression, with evidence that the pandemic has seen rates spike even further: 300 people a day are going to A&E departments because of feeling depressed, the NHS reported last week.

For many, the mainstay treatments offer limited benefit. According to the World Health Organization, around 30 per cent of people do not respond to existing treatments of antidepressant drugs, psychotherapy or electroconvulsive therapy. A recent study of antidepressants, published in the New England Journal of Medicine, found that even after two years of treatment, six out of 10 who felt well enough to stop taking them suffered a relapse within a year, compared to a relapse of four in 10 among those who continued their pills.

There remain concerns about side effects, too. Various studies have found links between long term use of selective serotonin reuptake inhibitors (SSRIs – the most commonly used antidepressants) and an increased risk of heart disease, strokes, obesity and type 2 diabetes, as well as the development of side effects such as sexual dysfunction. In older adults, they are associated with falls, fractures and a greater risk of bleeding.

The need for an alternative to prescription pills has never been greater – and a range of new antidepressant therapies are causing many to rethink depression and how we treat it.

Many are aimed at the estimated 12 to 20 per cent of treatment-resistant patients for whom all other approaches have failed. But they are also gaining traction among patients with more mild to moderate illness, who are concerned about the potential consequences of taking antidepressants over the course of years or even decades.

Dunning became so desperate for help with his depression that he contemplated undergoing electroconvulsive therapy, a last resort treatment still used for the most severe forms, where a mild electric current is passed through the brain to reset circuitry. In the end though, he opted to receive ketamine infusions at a private clinic in London. And for the first time in his life, he began to experience relief. 'It offered a pretty much instantaneous benefit,' he says. 'Since then I've found a cycle which works for me, I go regularly, but not every week, and I feel happy with my life.'

Ketamine and the psychedelic drug psilocybin – the active ingredient in magic mushrooms – are attracting growing attention for their potential benefits for mental health problems in recent years. Such is the evidence that some NHS trusts now offer ketamine treatment for severe depression, as a paid for service. Scientists are still not entirely sure how it works, but while SSRIs attempt to increase the levels of serotonin – a hormone involved in regulating mood – in the brain, ketamine is known to target another chemical called glutamate which is linked to a whole variety of mental illnesses. It is also thought to help repair damaged connections between cells involved in mood.

Like SSRIs, psilocybin also targets serotonin, but in a subtly different way. Psilocybin helps relax thoughts and emotions, which appears to help depression patients become more receptive to the benefits of psychotherapy.

'There's a lot of excitement about these new agents and I can understand why,' says Steven Marwaha, professor of psychiatry at the University of Birmingham. 'There's been a number of open label studies [where participants know about the treatment they are receiving] in which people who are having psychotherapy also have psilocybin, and it seems to have a positive effect, also one or two in the absence of psychotherapy, and there again seems to be a reduction of depressive symptoms.'

In one study last year, conducted by psychiatrists at the Karolinska Institute in Stockholm, 48 per cent of treatment-resistant depression patients, who had not responded to SSRIs, saw remission of their symptoms after ketamine treatment.

Prof Marwaha says the National Institute for Health and Care Excellence is currently considering approving a ketamine-based drug known as esketamine for use on the NHS. 'It seems to have a rapid, and fairly persistent effect on the treatment of depression,' says Marwaha.

But neither ketamine nor psilocybin are a complete panacea. These drugs do not work for all patients and concerns have been repeatedly raised about their side-effect profiles, which can include hallucinations and out-of-body experiences following treatment, as well as fluctuations in blood pressure.

Another area of research showing promise, with a lower risk of side-effects, is brain stimulation. This month, scientists at the University of California San Francisco reported on a woman with severe depression whose symptoms had been dramatically alleviated by an electrical brain implant. Their finding was hailed as a landmark achievement in the drive for new treatments in mental health. The patient, known only as Sarah, said that wearing the device for a year had 'kept depression at bay, allowing me to return to my best self and rebuild a life worth living'.

Previous brain stimulation devices tested for depression have had mixed results. This is thought to be because most devices only stimulate one area of the brain, while depression involves different brain regions in different people.

In the latest study, the researchers identified a specific pattern of brain activity which indicated the onset of the patient's negative feelings, and embedded a deep brain stimulation device – equivalent to a pacemaker for the brain – which is designed to recognise that pattern and neutralise it by administering a mild electric pulse.

'The device has learned what depressive-like electrical activity looks like in the brain of the depressed patient,' explained James Potash, psychiatrist-in-chief at Johns Hopkins Medicine in Baltimore. 'When it sees that pattern, it fires for six seconds to disrupt and reset the bad pattern. Then it turns off. The patient doesn't sense anything has happened. It can do this up to 300 times a day.'

As it is such a personalised therapy, Potash says that it remains to be seen whether it can be applied to the wider patient population.

What about tech? The pandemic and its impact on mental health have seen people turning in their droves to digital apps and platforms, encompassing everything from mood tracking apps to chatbot psychologists. There are now more than 10,000 different mental health apps on the market, according to the World Economic Forum. But while many claim to be useful at diagnosing depression or improving symptoms and self-management, there is scant independent evidence of their efficacy. The industry is also almost entirely unregulated, meaning there is no standardised quality of virtual therapists, a source of concern to many psychiatrists.

'There's very little trial evidence, which in effect means that no one's investigated the harms of these apps,' says Prof Marwaha. 'There is some evidence that if you're rating your mood constantly over the course of a week, then you see at the end of the week that it's pretty low, that may make you feel more low.'

With long waiting lists for talking therapies on the NHS, therapy apps remain a cheap and accessible alternative, though it may prove that they are only useful for the very mildest forms of the disease. Research has previously shown psychotherapy is most effective for mild-moderate depression when used in combination with SSRIs.

Traditional antidepressants remain a lifeline for many patients. Doctors stress that it is important that patients do not switch to other therapies before first consulting with their psychiatrist. 'Trials have shown that antidepressants are effective to an extent in reducing relapse,' says Tony Kendrick, professor of primary care at the University of Southampton. 'Most of them cost a few pounds a month, so someone can be on them for a year for £30 and it costs that much for an hour of psychotherapy. So clearly they're cost effective to the NHS.'

Nevertheless, with such a range of different therapies being explored, there is increasing hope that depression will become a far more manageable condition.

'There have been people who have been struggling with depression for all of their life, and we really hope that with all this research taking place, many of them will get better,' says Carmine Pariante, professor of biological psychiatry at King's College London. 'We will have more tools available in future than ever before.'

*18 October 2021*

# Mark Cavendish keen to use his battle with depression to help others

The 36-year-old Manxman had a memorable 2021 when he won four stages at the Tour de France.

*By Ian Parker*

Mark Cavendish wants to use his experience of battling depression to help others who may be suffering from mental health problems.

The 36-year-old enjoyed a stunning renaissance in 2021 as he won four stages of the Tour de France – his first since 2016 – to equal Eddy Merckx's record of 34, earning a nomination for Comeback of the Year in the Laureus World Sports Awards.

The wins were all the more special given Cavendish had been dogged by injury and illness for several seasons, struggles which left him clinically depressed.

The Manxman has admitted he previously believed that 'depression was an excuse' but he now wants to talk about his own experience to help others.

'I was somebody before who didn't really believe mental health problems were a thing,' he said. 'The irony that I suffered was such a good thing because it meant I could personally talk about the fact it is real.'

Cavendish's problems began soon after he won four stages of the 2016 Tour before withdrawing early in order to compete on the track at the Rio Olympics, where he won omnium silver.

The following year he suffered from the Epstein-Barr virus, initially misdiagnosed, while a series of crashes added to his problems.

A rider who had made winning look routine took only two victories between 2017 and 2020 – fearing his career was over.

'I went from being the best in the world to one of the worst overnight,' he said.

'I was misdiagnosed and mishandled by people I trusted in an old team and it pretty much wiped out everything physically I had worked for, and along with that came mental health problems...

'I know there's still a stigma about it. I know it's not taken seriously. If I didn't take it seriously I know a lot more people don't take it seriously. But I'm fortunate to have a platform to talk about it, to talk from personal experience and that has a lot more power.

'If you think you'll never get it, if you think, 'Oh, I'm strong', it's not about being strong or weak in the head. It's an illness. It's chemical. It's something you can't control.

'In every interview I do I'll talk about my problems because if one person can take something from it then it's worth it. I'll talk about it because I know how damaging it can be not just for your life but other people around you.'

Cavendish has previously spoken about the vital role his wife Peta played in his comeback, pushing him when he could not push himself, encouraging him when his belief wavered, and his answer when asked what has been his greatest win is telling.

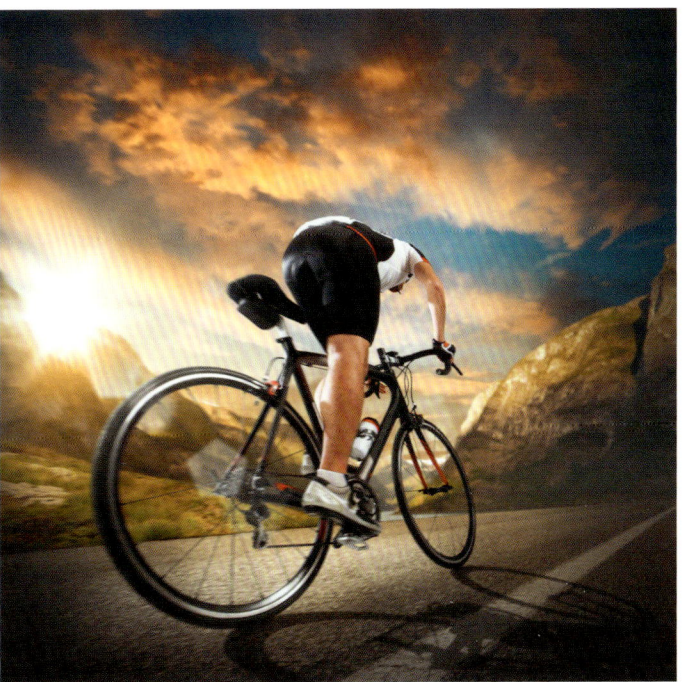

'That I still have a family after what my job takes from me, after my life was turned upside down with physical and mental illness,' he said. 'That I still have my family is the biggest victory I could ever hope for. That's for sure.'

Last year's Tour was one of the great sporting fairytales.

Months before he gave a tearful post-race interview, admitting he feared his career was over. But then he was offered a one-year, minimum wage deal with Deceuninck-QuickStep – now Quick-Step Alpha Vinyl – and when Sam Bennett suffered a knee injury, the door opened for an unexpected return to the Tour.

Even then, few would have foreseen the four stage wins that followed.

'Last year I got asked a lot about stars aligning, but there's a difference between stars aligning and you going to every single star and burning your hands to pull it into line,' he said.

'As a sportsperson I can weep about my hard times, but that's what makes a comeback – when you've had hard times. I'm fortunate that a comeback means I've got something back.

'A lot of people are in a position where they're still fighting. All I can say is, don't give up.'

*18 February 2022*

---

The above information is reprinted with kind permission from *The Independent*.
© independent.co.uk 2022

**www.independent.co.uk**

# Best evidence suggests antidepressants aren't very effective in kids and teens. What can be done instead?

An article from *The Conversation*.

By Sarah Hetric, Associate Professor of Youth Mental Health, University of Auckland, Joanne McKenzie, Associate Professor, Biostatistics Unit, School of Public Health and Preventive Medicine, Monash University, Nick Meader, Research Fellow, Centre for Reviews and Dissemination, University of York & Sally Merry, Professor and Cure Kids Duke Family Chair in Child and Adolescent Mental Health, University of Auckland

Even before COVID-19 lockdowns, school closures and strict social distancing, depression was on the rise in children and teenagers around the globe.

By the age of 19, around 25% of adolescents are estimated to have experienced a depressive episode. By the age of 30, this figure grows to 53%.

A number of studies point to an increasing use of antidepressants in young people.

So, what do we now know about how well antidepressants work in children and young people?

Our new Cochrane review, published today, found that on average, antidepressants led to only small improvements in depression symptoms compared with placebo in children and adolescents (ranging in age from six to 18 years old).

## Antidepressants shouldn't be the first port of call

Our findings highlight antidepressants are no panacea for depression in young people. The small improvements might be so small as to not be very noticeable to the individual person. What's more, we can't say to any one young person whether antidepressants will definitely improve their symptoms.

But it's critical to note there are multiple and complex pathways that lead to the distress and demoralisation that are key in depression.

Different people's responses to antidepressants are therefore quite specific, and young people may experience anything from marked improvement to deterioration.

Another important finding is that antidepressants are associated with an increased risk of suicidal thinking and self-harm.

These are not necessarily new findings, but they represent the best evidence we have so far. They remain a key consideration for GPs and other health professionals who are considering medications for children and young people.

What is new is our findings on how different antidepressants compare with each other. Many current guidelines recommend fluoxetine as the only first-line medication that should be tried. This is commonly sold under the brand name Prozac.

Fluoxetine is what's called a "selective serotonin reuptake inhibitor" (SSRI). Serotonin is a neurotransmitter in the brain linked to positive emotions. After it's used by nerve cells, serotonin is reabsorbed, which is known as "reuptake". These types of antidepressants work by blocking the reuptake of serotonin, therefore increasing its availability to pass messages between nerve cells.

Our review shows three other antidepressants, including sertraline, escitalopram, and duloxetine, had similar effects to fluoxetine. Though, there's the caveat that all of these led to only small reductions in depression on average.

However, this finding may extend treatment options for young people with depression. For example, one of these antidepressants may suit one person better than another in terms of side-effects experienced, and the time it takes to work or to wash out of the system.

## What other options are there?

Against a backdrop of a global pandemic, there's a risk we may start to consider depression as the "norm", passing it over as a given or as insignificant.

But as those with depression, and their parents, families and friends know, depression is anything but. It impacts every facet of life and is often accompanied by a fear it may never improve.

Depression varies substantially between people with multiple factors at play, so it's important a range of support and treatments are available for people.

Antidepressants have been, and will remain, only one of many options for young people with depression. Guidelines continue to highlight that antidepressants should not be the first port of call.

When used, they should be used in combination with evidence-based talking therapy, the most common being cognitive behavioural therapy (CBT), and there must be a commitment to ensure close monitoring of their impact.

There's a range of ways in which young people can and need to be supported. There's good evidence for regular physical activity, good nutrition, and adequate sleep. Support from family, schools and the broader community is also important.

A decision to use antidepressants should be on the basis of shared decision-making. This refers to conversations where the risks and benefits of all treatment options are described to the young person, and their family, who are then meaningfully involved in making the decision.

If the decision is made to use an antidepressant, it's critical to ensure health professionals conduct regular (weekly at first) checks on depression symptoms and adverse effects. This is particularly important in terms of monitoring the emergence of suicidal thinking and self-harm.

Treatment with an antidepressant should be in the context of talking therapy, and a holistic approach to well-being.

Ensuring access to support and treatment and conveying a sense of hope is crucial.

*24 May 2021*

The above information is reprinted with kind permission from The Conversation.
© 2010-2022, The Conversation Trust (UK) Limited

www.theconversation.com

# You can't control the headlines but here's some stuff you can control

It's been a pretty overwhelming time, with one wave of bad news after the next. There's uncertainty over where things are heading in Ukraine, the rising cost of living, climate change worries and how we adapt to living with covid – things feel shit right now, so we've put together some stuff that might help. However bad things are, we're here, united.

The last couple of years have been weird, filled with lockdowns, worrying headlines and scientists pointing at scary graphs. It's been a tough, anxiety-inducing time. Then, when things started to get back to normal, a load of other shit hit the fan.

So it's not surprising we've got used to waiting for bad news and when things are out of our control, it's easy to feel helpless. While we can't control a lot of what's going on, here's some stuff you can control.

## United against doomscrolling

It's good to stay in-the-know about what's going on in the world, but sometimes you need a break from bad news.

As humans, we're hardwired to pay attention to the bad stuff, so even when we're mindlessly scrolling through Instagram, our brains are subconsciously sucking up all those negative vibes. It can really take its toll on our mental wellbeing, impact how we sleep, our eating habits, and just leave us feeling a bit meh. So if the headlines are making your head hurt, try these:

- Limit the time you spend with your head in the news – a quick 30 minutes or less on the headlines is probably enough.
- Balance bad news with positive news, or just some lighter content (there's nothing quite like otter taps to cheer you up).
- Avoid checking your phone right before bed if things feel too much and remember, you control your social feed. Unfollow, temporarily block, or just turn on focus-mode if you need a break.
- Sometimes news gets muddled or messed with as it travels down the grapevine, so if you want to fact check that story your auntie shared on Facebook, try a looking on a fact-checking site such as fullfact.org.

### United against ignoring your worries

Allowing yourself a moment to scream into a pillow, or just sit and reflect is okay.

It's fine to have a lot of different feelings about everything going on, but worries can quickly stack up and take over. We know it's not as simple as saying 'don't worry', but there are ways you can minimise the worries that seep into things like your work or down time:

- Mates are amazing medicine, so put in some time for a call, or meet up at your local to put the world to rights.
- It sounds a bit weird, but schedule in time to worry. In that time, write down all the things which are playing on your mind – whether that's on paper or the Notes bit of your phone. It doesn't matter how big or small they are, just get it all out.
- It's easy to get stuck in a whirlpool of what-ifs, but these are normally the worries you can't control. Try to let them go.

## United against feeling helpless

We might not have a hold of the world's steering wheel, but that doesn't mean there aren't small things we can do to feel more empowered.

There's always going to be a level of uncertainty in life, but that doesn't mean we have to leave everything up to chance. Taking back a bit of control, can make us feel a bit better about the things going on in the world right now.

- That might mean giving meat-free Monday a go, or donating to a charity that's helping to do something about the things you care about.
- Life's getting increasingly expensive, so If money-pressures are mounting up, look at cancelling subscriptions, eating at home more, or walking/car-sharing to work.
- If things are feeling overwhelming, try writing down a to-do list. Crossing things out can help you feel more in control.
- Get out and do something you enjoy, whether that's playing football with your mates or sprinting off some stress at your local park.

## United against feeling alone

When everything around you feels like a lot, it can seem like you're on your own, but CALM's got your back.

No matter how heavy it all feels, you don't have to struggle alone – life can be miserable, but it doesn't have to be. Whatever's on your mind, whether it's the world's or your own problems, reaching out can really help.

*10 March 2022*

The above information is reprinted with kind permission from CALM
© CALM 2022

www.thecalmzone.net

# How to cope with bad news

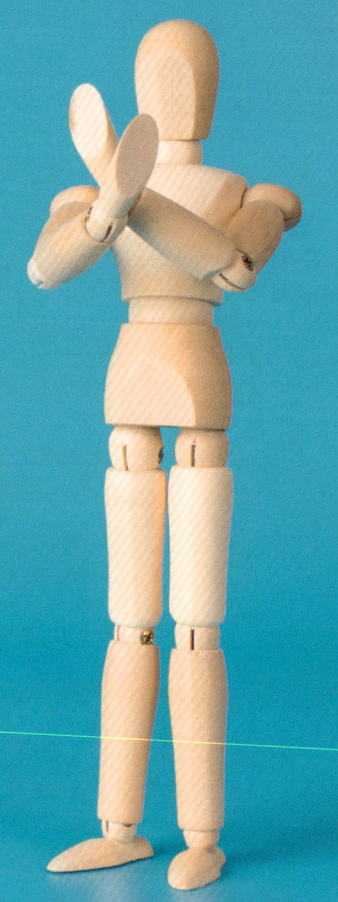

War in Ukraine, the spiralling cost of living and the climate crisis are putting a strain on people's mental heath. We spoke to experts about how to cope with bad news, this is what they said.

By Robin Eveleigh

### 1. Put the kettle on

The quintessentially British response of 'putting the kettle on' in troubled times might seem like a quaint notion, but the naturally calming effects of tea – which is shown to lower levels of the stress hormone cortisol – makes it a sage place to start.

### 2. Manage your media diet

The temptation to doomscroll through social media or watch rolling news may be strong in times of crisis, but is best avoided. The link between such behaviour and poor mental health has been proven by studies.

That's not to say don't engage – it's important to know what's going on – but limiting news consumption, rather than gorging on it all day, is advisable.

Offsetting the doom with uplifting stories is also vital. The World Health Organization recommended that people do this during the pandemic, but the advice applies to any crisis.

### 3. Take positive action

In the face of bad news – and there's a lot of it about – it's easy to feel overwhelmed by a sense of powerlessness.

Harley Street trauma expert Olivia James suggests focusing on positive action you could take to break out of stasis. 'Even if it's just a small thing,' she says. 'Do something rather than just taking in all the bad news and feeling more and more immobilised by it all.'

Cognitive behaviour therapist Navit Schechter agrees. 'Worrying is a thought process which can quickly spin out of control. Focus on the moment – think about what you can do to offer support.'

### 4. Breathe deeply

Taking a deep breath is another classic bit of bad news advice, but – much like tea drinking – there's some science behind it.

Neuro-linguisting programming trainer Andy Coley says a fight-or-flight response in stressful situations is great for rapid response to an emergency – but not so great if your gas bill sends you into a tailspin.

'Deep and slow belly breathing triggers part of the nervous system, which lowers cortisol and adrenaline, and raises oxytocin and dopamine,' explains Coley. 'Oxytocin is the 'chemical of love' – it floods your body with good feelings. And while you might not fall in love with that gas bill, you will at least be able to think more clearly, with some perspective.'

### 5. Activate your brain for 'aha' solutions

Marilyn Devonish overcame suicidal depression to become a certified coach and therapist, and has 21 years' experience working in the trauma field. 'Continual bad news almost tipped me over the edge,' she says.

Devonish is another advocate of pausing for breath. 'If you don't oxygenate your brain, it will shut down to some extent, and that often means you are – quite literally – not thinking straight.'

She says activating the brain to move past bad news and towards a solution, or positive response, is key. 'Sometimes that next step is to just sit with it and feel whatever you're feeling,' she explains. 'But if you tell your brain what you want, it will do what it can to help you. Out of the blue you'll come up with one of those 'aha' moments.'

### 6. Mindfulness over matter

In similar vein, former NHS GP Nicola Harker says we're hardwired to read the worst into bad news, and often leap to unhelpful assumptions.

'We're wired for survival rather than happiness,' says Harker, who is now working as a coach with a focus on mindful self-compassion.

'Notice how your brain goes to worse case scenarios and notice the narrative that is running in your mind. The brain loves to go to 'all or nothing', but the reality is usually somewhere in between. You can find comfort, connection, even joy in difficult times. With a growth mindset, you can come through terrible situations.'

### 7. Sleep on it

Grim news can often precipitate rash decision making, turning your bad tidings into catastrophe. Clinical psychotherapist Tania Taylor recommends taking time out.

'It's easy to jump into taking action that you'll later regret,' she says. 'If you can, sleep on it. When we sleep, our memories from the day are processed and moved from our emotional to our narrative mind. We can then think about them and make decisions using the intelligent part of our brain rather than our 'fight or flight' limbic system.'

### 8. Shake it out

Sylvia Tillmann is a provider of Tension and Trauma Releasing Exercises. She says our innate bodily reaction of shaking or trembling in immediate response to trauma and bad news should be encouraged rather than suppressed.

'We've been socialised out of it,' she laments. 'We perceive tremors as weakness, something embarrassing, or even as illness.

'Shaking after a stressful or traumatic event is good for us as tremors enable a disrupted nervous system to bring body and mind back into balance, finalising the stress response. It's an innate and very natural reaction. We should trust our body wisdom.'

### 9. Prepare for aftershock

Conversely, our response to bad news may not always be as instant, or as visible, as a case of the shakes. Geraldine Joaquim, a clinical hypnotherapist, advises being prepared for a delayed reaction.

'It might seem that you take it all in in the moment, but afterwards is when maybe the tears or emotion come because it just takes a little while to filter through,' she says. 'Recognise that you don't always have to keep soldiering on, and allow yourself some self-compassion.'

### 10. Talk about it

Finally, psychologist and wellbeing consultant Lee Chambers advises reaching out to friends and family for support, or finding professional help.

'It's easy to internalise things and fall into your own unhealthy coping mechanisms,' he says. 'Recognise the value of positive social support when you've had bad news – expressing the negative emotions that come with it enables us to take ownership of them, and begins the process of being more self-compassionate and kind to ourselves.'

*8 March 2022*

---

The above information is reprinted with kind permission from Postive.News
© Positive News 2022

**www.positive.news**

# Talking therapies

Talking therapies can help you deal with negative thoughts and feelings and make positive changes.

Talking therapy involves talking to a trained professional about your thoughts, feelings and behaviour. Describing what's going on in your head and how that makes you feel can help you notice any patterns you may want to change. It can help you work out where your negative feelings and ideas come from and why they are there.

Understanding all this can help you make positive changes, take greater control of your life and improve your confidence.

This page uses the word 'talking therapy', but you may also hear it referred to as talking treatment, counselling, therapy, psychotherapy or psychological therapy.

## Who can benefit from talking therapy?

Talking therapy can help with:

- difficult life events such as bereavement or redundancy
- relationship problems
- events from your past that still cause you distress – consciously or unconsciously
- difficult feelings such as anger, shame or low self-esteem
- mental health problems
- some long-term physical health conditions.

It doesn't have to be a last resort or something you turn to in a crisis. If you think you could do with talking to someone in a safe space who won't judge you, then it's ok to try it.

## How do I know which kind of therapy is right for me?

There are many different approaches when it comes to therapy. Therapists may train in one approach or use a number of different methods. Some use specialist techniques – for example, an art therapist would use art to help you explore your feelings. Others offer specialist treatment for specific issues such as addictions or eating disorders.

It can be easy to be overwhelmed by the number of different types of talking therapy out there. Don't let that put you off. We go through some different types below, but the most important thing is the relationship you have with your therapist. Trusting them and feeling comfortable opening up means you will get the most from your sessions, no matter what approach they use.

## Different types of talking therapy

There are many different types of talking therapy, although your choice may be limited depending on where and how you access it.

The National Institute for Health and Care Excellence (NICE) recommends certain therapies for certain problems, but other therapies might work for you just as well.

Here are some of the main kinds of talking therapy.

## Cognitive behavioural therapy (CBT)

This looks at how your thoughts and beliefs affect your feelings and behaviour. By changing how you react to your thoughts (for example, challenging negative thoughts) and how you behave (for example, trying new activities), you can start to feel better.

### What's unique about it?

CBT tends to be short-term – often between six and 12 sessions – and takes a more structured approach than other therapies. It looks at specific problems rather than how you feel more generally. You'll often have tasks to do between sessions such as keeping a diary or practising the skills you've learned in therapy.

### What can it help with?

CBT can help with a range of problems including depression, anxiety, obsessive compulsive disorder, managing long-term illnesses, eating disorders, post-traumatic stress and schizophrenia.

*'CBT was amazing - it was so simple. My diagnosis is bipolar disorder and I had very low self-esteem and lack of confidence in my future. I had about 15 sessions over a year. The psychologist showed me how to notice what I was thinking and then how I felt afterwards, and to realise you can choose your own thoughts. I thought they were just random thoughts there to make my life a misery. But I learnt that at any time I could stop and say: 'Why am I thinking that?'*

*'I had a CBT therapist but I think she probably used lots of different things - in fact it didn't feel like she was 'using' anything - it felt like a natural process rather than anything very medical or clinical.'*

## Dialectical behaviour therapy (DBT)

DBT is an adapted form of cognitive behavioural therapy (CBT) that can help people who experience emotions very intensely. It teaches you how to live in the moment, cope with stress, regulate your emotions and improve your relationships.

### What's unique about it?

'Dialectical' comes from the idea that bringing together two opposites – acceptance and change – can make a bigger difference than either one alone. Accepting yourself and changing your behaviour might sound like a contradiction, but your therapist will help you understand how this can bring about positive shifts in your life.

### What can it help with?

It was originally designed to treat borderline personality disorder but now it's also used for eating disorders, addiction, depression and problems such as self-harm or suicidal feelings.

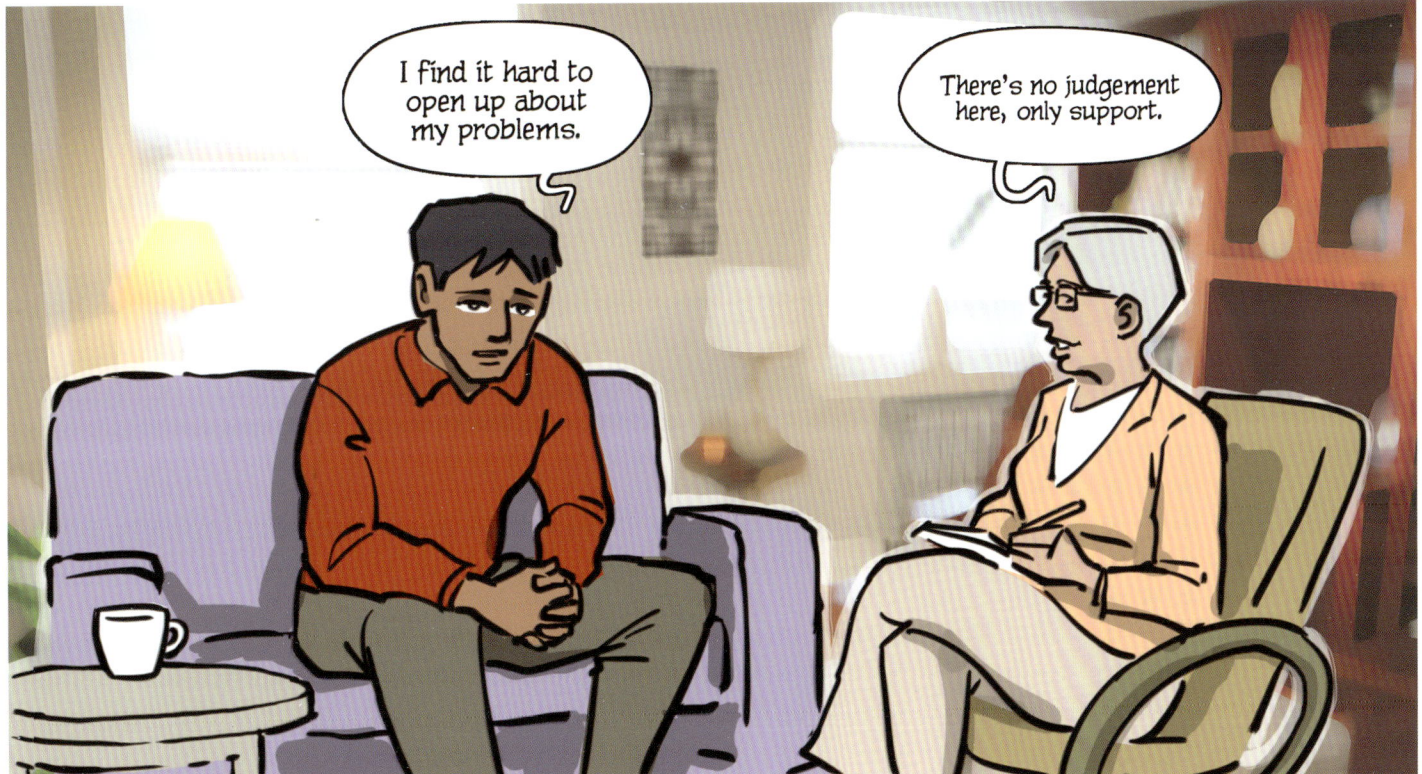

### Psychodynamic therapy

Psychodynamic therapy explores how your childhood experiences and unconscious mind influences your current thoughts, feelings, relationships and behaviour. Your therapist may use techniques such as:

- free association – where you talk freely about whatever is on your mind, no matter how silly or illogical it might seem, to let your true feelings come to the surface
- transference – where feelings you experienced in other relationships, especially from childhood, are unconsciously projected onto your therapist. By recognising this, you can start to understand these feelings and past relationships
- interpretation – your therapist will sometimes offer a new perspective on what you're talking about, aiming to help you broaden your self-awareness and self-knowledge.

### What's unique about it?

Psychodynamic therapy focuses more on your past and on your unconscious mind – the feelings and thoughts that you're not aware of but that affect your choices and actions in the present day. It's often relatively long-term, lasting from several months to many years.

### What is it helpful for?

Depression, anxiety, post-traumatic stress, long-term physical health problems, eating disorders and addictions. NICE recommends psychodynamic therapy for people experiencing depression alongside other complex illnesses.

*'I was quite severely depressed as a teenager. I tried various antidepressants and some CBT-based stuff, but nothing was helping. Finally, my GP suggested that I try psychotherapy at my local mental health unit.'*

*'At first I was sceptical. I couldn't see how sitting in a room with a stranger was going to help. I was quite a nightmare, trying to prove to my therapist and myself that the therapy would fail. But with psychodynamic therapy, the therapist is prepared to sit and wait out that part with you. She started helping me link the way I was thinking, feeling and behaving to what might have gone on when I was younger and that really made sense.'*

### Humanistic therapy

Humanistic therapy lets you explore your whole self rather than just specific problems. It aims to help you grow, live your life to the full and be true to yourself. Your therapist will offer you empathy, warmth and genuineness to help you make these changes.

Person-centred therapy, Gestalt therapy and transactional analysis are all examples of humanistic therapy. The British Association for Counselling and Psychotherapy (BACP) has more information about them.

### What's unique about it?

Humanistic therapy focuses on all of you. It's based on the belief that we are all capable of growth but that life experiences may have blocked us from reaching our potential. Your therapist can help you identify and remove those blocks.

### What is it helpful for?

Anxiety, depression, obsessive-compulsive disorder (OCD), post-traumatic stress disorder (PTSD), personality disorders and more. A humanistic therapist will work with any issue causing difficulties in your life.

*'I was referred to a unit that deals with people who turn to alcohol because of psychological problems. I was in a state of constant panic and had been drinking to keep those feelings at bay. There wasn't a set formula to the sessions. We'd just go and get a cup of coffee and I'd talk about what was bothering me. With person-centred*

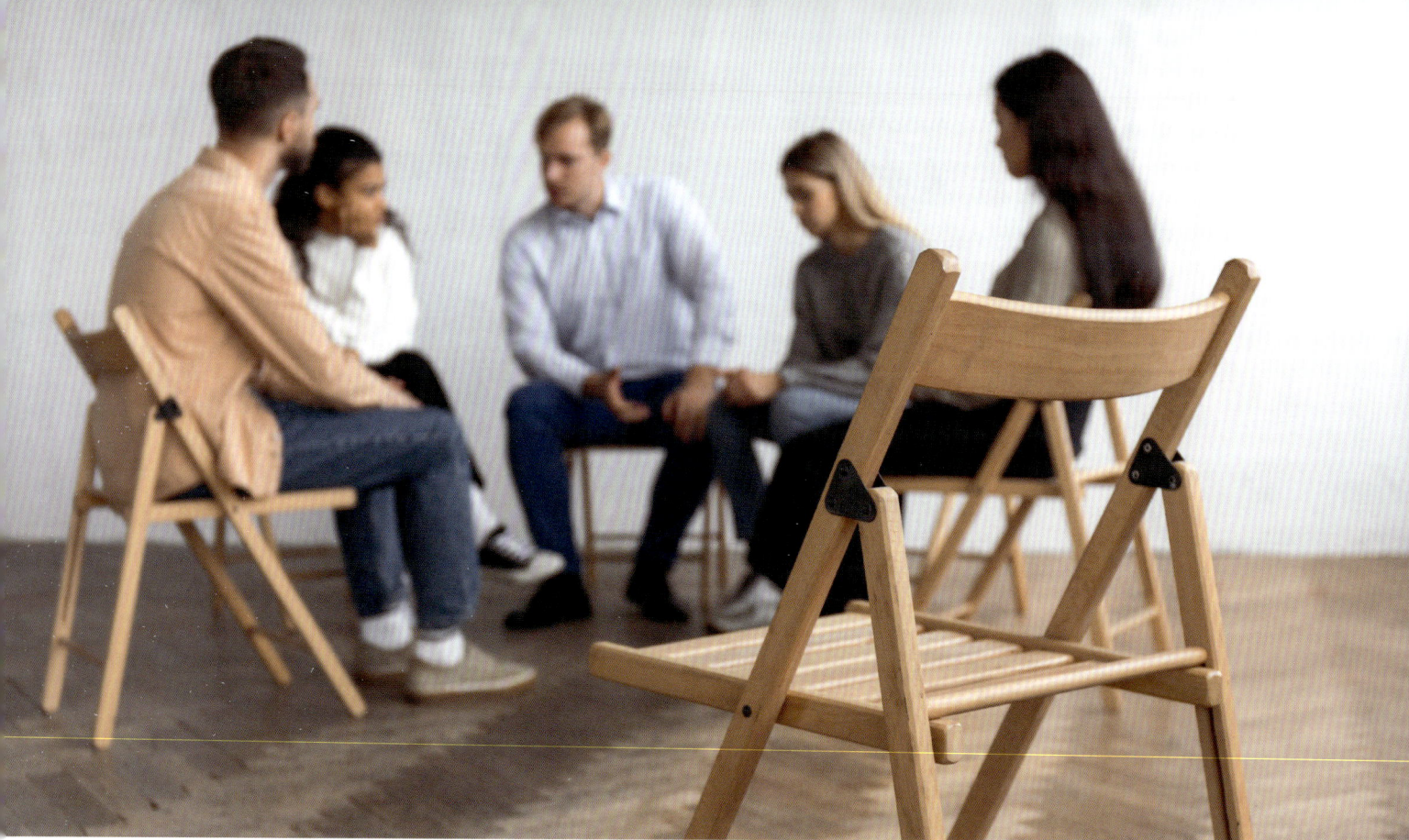

*counselling the therapist steers you through finding out more about yourself and developing confidence.'*

### How do I find a therapist?
You can find a therapist in different ways, although not all types of therapy will be available everywhere.

### Through the NHS
Your GP or another health professional may refer you to a qualified therapist or you can self-refer if you live in England. The therapy will be provided free on the NHS.

In many places there are long waiting lists and you may not have much choice who you see.

National Institute for Health and Care Excellence(NICE) advises which treatments doctors should prescribe. NICE recommends certain therapies for certain problems and these may be easier to get on the NHS than others.

### Go private
If you can afford it, you can choose to pay for your own therapy. Therapists may charge anything from £35 an hour and more depending on where you live, although some offer reductions to people on a low income.

To find a private therapist, it's a good idea to search via a website that only lists therapists who are registered with a professional body such as:

- the British Association for Counselling and Psychotherapy (BACP) for all kinds of therapists
- Counselling Directory for all kinds of therapists
- the Online CBT Register for cognitive behavioural therapy (CBT) practitioners
- Pink Therapy for therapists with LGBTQI+ experience
- the Black, African and Asian Therapy Network (BAATN) for therapists of Black, African, South Asian and Caribbean heritage.

### Through your place of work or education
Some workplaces have Employee Assistance Programmes (EAPs) which may offer a limited number of free therapy sessions. Many colleges and universities offer free therapy services.

### Other organisations
Some charities and community organisations offer talking therapies free or at low cost, sometimes by using trainees. Ask your GP if they know anywhere local, contact local counselling training centres, or try one of the following.

- Your local Mind or Rethink may offer talking therapy.
- Anxiety UK offers reduced rate therapy.
- The British Psychotherapy Association offers low-cost intensive therapy. You need to make a two year minimum commitment.
- Cruse Bereavement Care offers bereavement counselling through its local branches.
- Sign Health offers free therapy to deaf people via sign language, lip reading or deaf-blind communication.

### What happens in talking therapy?
Sessions usually last 50 minutes and take place at regular, planned times. They can be face-to-face, on the phone or online. How often you see your therapist and how many sessions you have will depend on the type of therapy you're having and your personal circumstances.

You might see a therapist on your own, in a group, as a couple or as a family.

*'In group therapy you don't just talk about yourself, you're listening to other people - that takes the burden off your problems. You realise you're not the only one.'*

During a session you might talk generally about how you're feeling or you might go through specific exercises, depending on your therapist's approach. What you talk about could include your childhood, your relationships, past and present life events or stressful situations, for example.

Your therapist will listen to you without judging you and help you explore your thoughts and feelings. They won't tell you what to do but will help you understand yourself better and think about the changes you may want to make.

Talking therapies are not therapies that are 'done' to you by someone else. You play an active part. That can be empowering at a time when you may feel you have lost control over part of your life. If you're determined to get the most from your therapy, it's more likely to work.

You need to be honest with yourself in therapy and that can be difficult. It may mean facing up to your fears, recalling distressing memories or talking about intimate topics and private thoughts and feelings. Think about whether you're ready to open up and talk to your therapist if you're feeling overwhelmed. Sessions should always go at your pace so you don't feel rushed.

### How do I choose a therapist?

You may already have questions to ask yourself or your therapist. Here are some to consider.

### Questions you could ask yourself before you choose a therapist

- What kind of therapy might suit me?
- How much time and money do I have for therapy?
- Do I want a particular therapist – eg a man or woman, someone who shares my racial background or sexuality, someone my own age?

### Questions you may want to ask a therapist

- What are your qualifications?
- What other training have you done?
- Do you belong to a professional organisation?
- What experience do you have of working with people with my particular issue?
- What happens at a typical session?
- How many sessions would I have?
- What is the cost for each session? Do you offer any reductions?

When you meet a therapist for the first time (sometimes called an assessment), they will be working out if they can help you. That's your chance to find out about the therapist too. The British Association for Counselling and Psychotherapy (BACP) has an information sheet on what happens in your first session.

### Ask yourself:

- Do I feel comfortable talking to them?
- Would I be able to trust and work with them?
- What's my gut feeling about them?

It might take a few tries before you find a therapist you connect with. Take your time to find someone who feels right so that you can get the most from your sessions.

### What makes a good therapist?

Your relationship with your therapist is really important. A good therapist will listen to you, have your best interests at heart and help you learn how to change. They will check you're getting what you want from therapy and refer you to someone else if they can't help with your particular issue.

*What I found really good was being able to talk about what was happening and have someone who was listening - she was really good at giving me space, listening to what had happened and discussing what might have caused it - not in a deep way but trying to help me piece the whole picture together.*

A good therapist concentrates on you – what is important in your life, what you want to achieve, what steps you could take to get there. They shouldn't tell you what to do. Your therapist may be highly trained and very experienced, but you are the expert on you.

Remember therapy is a two-way process. If you have any questions, ask them. A good therapist will help you deal with your worries and work out how you will manage when therapy comes to an end.

### What if I'm not happy with my therapist?

It can take time to build a relationship with your therapist and start to open up. You may feel sad or frustrated after sessions at times depending on what you've talked about. But if you're not happy with how the sessions are going, you can:

- talk to your therapist to try and resolve any problems
- ask your therapist if they can try a different approach
- go back to your GP or referral service to ask if you can see someone else
- find another private therapist.

### If you need to make a complaint

If you have a serious concern about your therapist, you can make a complaint.

You can contact the professional body your therapist is registered with and follow their complaints procedure. You can ask your therapist who they're registered with or see if it's mentioned in your contract, if you have one. For example, you can complain about a BACP member or a UKCP member by following the steps on their websites.

The BACP has a 'get help with counselling concerns' service you can contact by phone or email. They can help you make sense of what you think has gone wrong and work out your next steps.

*September 2021*

> The above information is reprinted with kind permission from the Mental Health Foundation
> © 2022. All Rights Reserved
>
> www.mentalhealth.org.uk

# Key Facts

- Globally, it is estimated that 5.0% of adults suffer from depression. (page 2)

- More women are affected by depression than men. (page 2)

- Although there are known, effective treatments for mental disorders, more than 75% of people in low- and middle-income countries receive no treatment. (page 2)

- Depression results from a complex interaction of social, psychological, and biological factors. (page 3)

- Over the period 21 July to 15 August 2021: Younger adults and women were more likely to experience some form of depression, with around 1 in 3 (32%) women aged 16 to 29 years experiencing moderate to severe depressive symptoms, compared with 20% of men of the same age. (page 6) Over the period 21 July to 15 August 2021: Of adults experiencing some form of depression, almost three-quarters (74%) reported that the coronavirus pandemic was affecting their well-being; this compared with around one in three (32%) adults with no or mild depressive symptoms. (page 6)

- A 2020 survey revealed that around 22% of UK adults have experienced job-related burnout. In fact, in August 2020, over 27,000 people worldwide searched the term 'burnout symptoms'. (page 8)

- The World Health Organization officially recognised 'burn-out' as a 'syndrome' in 2019, but only in an occupational context. It will be included in the 11th edition of the International Classification of Diseases (ICD-11) which takes effect in January 2022. Despite this, it isn't currently included in the Diagnostic and Statistical Manual of Mental Disorders (DSM-5). (page 8)

- Memory problems aren't discussed as widely as other symptoms. We know that cognitive impairments are common in depression. In fact, up to three in five people with depression may experience them. (page 12)

- The most commonly prescribed antidepressants, selective serotonin reuptake inhibitors (SSRI) and serotonergic-noradrenergic reuptake inhibitors (SNRI), are also associated with improvements in planning, decision-making and reasoning – though these findings are mixed, and may not work as well for older people (page 13)

- When we have depression, parts of our brain can shrink. (page 14)

- Cortisol is a hormone that's released when we're stressed. In the short-term, it's usually helpful. But when we live with long-term stress, for example when living with depression, our cortisol levels remain high which can start to cause problems. (page 15)

- People whose sleep pattern goes against their natural body clock – meaning they are forced to go to bed and wake up earlier or later than they'd like – are more likely to have depression and lower levels of wellbeing, according to a study. (page 17)

- As many as 1.3 million cases of depression can be put down to the material conditions people live in. (page 22)

- Figures from the NHS Business Services Authority show more than 20 million antidepressants were prescribed between October and December 2020 – a 6% increase compared with the same three months in 2019. (page 28)

- In one study conducted in 2020 by psychiatrists at the Karolinska Institute in Stockholm, 48 per cent of treatment-resistant depression patients, who had not responded to SSRIs, saw remission of their symptoms after ketamine treatment. (page 30)

# Glossary

### Antidepressants

These include tricyclic antidepressants (TCAs), selective serotonin re-uptake inhibitors (SSRIs) and monoamine oxidase inhibitors (MAOIs). Antidepressants work by boosting one of more chemicals (neurotransimitters) in the nervous system, which may present in insufficient amounts during a depressive illness.

### Anxiety

Anxiety can be described as a feeling of fear, apprehension, tension and/or stress. Most people experience anxiety from time to time and this is a perfectly normal response to stress. However, some individuals suffer from anxiety disorders which cause them to experience symptoms such as intense, persistent fear or nervousness, panic attacks and hyperventilation.

### Bipolar disorder

Previously called manic depression, this illness is characterised by mood swings where periods of severe depression are balanced by periods of elation and over-activity (mania).

### Burnout

Burnout is most commonly spoken of in work-related terms. It occurs when things have gone out of balance, and our stress and activity levels far outweigh the amount of rest we have.

### Clinical depression

Clinical depression means that a doctor has given you a diagnosis of depression.

### Cognitive behavioural therapy (CBT)

A psychological treatment which assumes that behavioural and emotional reactions are learned over a long period. A cognitive therapist will seek to identify the source of emotional problems and develop techniques to overcome them.

### Cyclothymia

You may be diagnosed with cyclothymia if you experience persistent and unstable moods. You may have periods of depression and periods of elation, but these periods may not be severe enough or long enough to be diagnosed as bipolar disorder.

### Depression

Someone is said to be significantly depressed, or suffering from depression, when feelings of sadness or misery don't go away quickly, and are so bad that they interfere with everyday life. Symptoms can also include low self-esteem and a lack of motivation.

### Dysthymia

This is when you are experiencing continuous mild depression that lasts for over 2 years. Also sometimes called persistent depressive disorder or chronic depression.

### Prenatal or postnatal depression

Prenatal depression occurs during pregnancy, it may also be called antenatal depression.

Postnatal depression occurs after becoming a parent. It can affect both men and women.

### Reactive depression

If your doctor thinks that your depression was triggered by difficult events in your life, such as divorce or money worries, they may say that it is reactive.

### Recurrent depressive disorder

If you've had at least 2 depressive episodes, your doctor might say that you have a recurrent depressive disorder. They may say that your current 'episode' is 'mild', 'moderate' or 'severe'.

### Seasonal affective disorder (SAD)

If you have SAD, you'll experience depression during particular seasons, or because of certain types of weather. You might find that your mood or energy levels drop when it gets colder or warmer, or notice changes in your sleeping or eating patterns.

It will affect you at the same time of year every year. It's most common during the winter.

### SSRIs

Selective serotonin uptake inhibitors. A medication widely used to treat depression and anxiety.

### Stress

Stress is the feeling of being under pressure. A little bit of pressure can be a good thing, helping to motivate you: however, too much pressure or prolonged pressure can lead to stress, which is unhealthy for the mind and body and can cause symptoms such as lack of sleep, loss of appetite and difficulty concentrating.

### Talking therapies

These involve talking and listening. Some therapists will aim to find the root of a sufferer's problem and help them deal with it, some will help to change behaviour and negative thoughts, while others simply offer support.

# Activities

- Think about times when you have felt down or depressed. Did you turn to any particular music or films that helped you feel a bit better? As a class, create a 'feel-good' list of songs, films, TV shows or books that have helped lift your spirits when you needed it.

## Brainstorming

- Brainstorm what you know about depression:
  - What is depression?
  - What is CBT?
  - What are antidepressants?
  - What is postnatal depression?

- Write a list of the reasons people might become depressed

- What kind of things can people do to cope with depression?

## Research

- Conduct some online research to find out what types of help are available in your area for people suffering with depression. You could look at helplines, self-help groups or charities for example. Do you think there is enough help out there?

- In pairs, do some research into the demographics of depression. Consider if depression affects people more or less depending on the following:
  - Age
  - Gender
  - Location
  - Line of work

- Write a short report on your findings and share with the rest of your class.

- In small groups, do some research in to how social media can affect a person's mood. Is it always negative? Compile a list of the negative and positive effects it can have on someone's mental health.

## Design

- Design a leaflet highlighting the issues of depression that young people are facing today. Your leaflet should offer help and advice on tackling these issues.

- Choose one of the articles in this book and create an illustration that highlights the key themes of the piece.

- Design a poster aimed at young people encouraging them to look after their mental health. Where would your display your poster?

## Oral

- Hold a class discussion on depression and low mood. What is the difference? Have you or your classmates suffered from either and if so, how did it feel? Does your school or college talk about and provide support with these issues?

- In pairs, role play one of the following situations:

- A student telling their friend that they are feeling very low about recent world events, and the friend's advice.

- An elderly person suffering with loneliness on the phone to a helpline, and the helpline counsellor's advice.

- A student telling a tutor they are feeling stressed and anxious about exams, and the tutor's advice.

- Choose one of the illustrations in this book, and in pairs, discuss what you think the artist was trying to portray with their image

## Reading/writing

- Write a diary entry from the point of view of someone who suffers from depression. Imagine how they would feel and what challenges they could face in their day-to-day life.

- Write a short definition of the each of the following types of depression:
  - Reactive depression
  - Bipolar disorder
  - Seasonal affective disorder (SAD)
  - Clinical depression

- Read the article *Mark Cavendish keen to use his battle with depression to help others* (page 31). Think about someone else you know of in the public eye who has spoken out about their own personal experience of depression. Write a short biography of that person and describe what you admire/find inspirational about them.

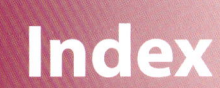

# Index

**A**
antidepressants 3, 5, 13, 16, 27, 29, 41
anxiety 11, 41
autistic burnout 8

**B**
bad news, coping with 34–35
Beck, A. 18–19
Beck Depression Inventory 18
bipolar disorder 3, 41
body clock 17
borderline personality disorder 36
boundaries 9
brain, and depression 14–16
British Association for Counselling and Psychotherapy (BACP) 39
burnout 8–10

**C**
Cavendish, M. 31
children and young people, and depression 3, 6, 20
Christmas, and depression 11
chronic depression 1
clinical depression 1, 41
cognitive behavioural therapy (CBT) 5, 18–19, 27, 36, 41
community mental health teams (CMHTs) 5
cortisol 15, 16
COVID-19, and depression 6–7, 11, 27
cyclothymia 1, 41

**D**
delusions 1
depression
   and the brain 14–16
   definition 41
   key facts 2–3
   recovery from 23–26
   statistics 2, 6
   treatments 3, 16, 18–19, 27, 36
   types 1
depressive episode 1–2
dialectical behaviour therapy (DBT) 36
doomscrolling 32–33
dysthymia 1, 41

**E**
electroconvulsive therapy (ECT) 16

**F**
Freud, S. 19

**G**
guilt 25

**H**
hallucinations 1
humanistic therapy 37–38

**I**
inflammation 15

**K**
ketamine 28–29

**M**
major depressive disorder (MDD) 14
manic depression 1
medication 3, 5, 13, 16, 27–30
memory 12
mood disorders 2–3

**O**
obsessive-compulsive disorder (OCD) 33, 37
Office for National Statistics, on depression 22

**P**
postnatal depression 1, 4–5, 41
postnatal psychosis 5
post-traumatic stress disorder (PTSD), 37
poverty, and depression 21–22
prenatal depression 1
psychodynamic therapy 36–37
psychosis 1
psychotherapy 16
   see also talking therapies
psychotic depression 1

**R**
reactive depression 1, 41
recurrent depressive disorder 1, 41

**S**
seasonal affective disorder (SAD) 1, 41
selective serotonin reuptake inhibitors (SSRIs) 3, 13, 29, 41
shame 25
sleep 35
   and depression 16–17
social media 32–34
stress 3, 8–9, 16, 32–34, 41
suicide 2

**T**
talking therapies 16, 27, 36–39, 41
   see also cognitive behavioural therapy (CBT)
transcranial magnetic stimulation (TMS) 16
tricyclic antidepressants (TCAs) 3

**W**
World Health Organization
   on depression 20
   Mental Health Action Plan 3

# Acknowledgements

The publisher is grateful for permission to reproduce the material in this book. While every care has been taken to trace and acknowledge copyright, the publisher tenders its apology for any accidental infringement or where copyright has proved untraceable. The publisher would be pleased to come to a suitable arrangement in any such case with the rightful owner.

The material reproduced in **issues** books is provided as an educational resource only. The views, opinions and information contained within reprinted material in **issues** books do not necessarily represent those of Independence Educational Publishers and its employees.

## Images

Cover image courtesy of iStock. All other images courtesy Freepik, Pixabay & Unsplash.

## Illustrations

Simon Kneebone: pages 15, 18 & 32. Angelo Madrid: pages 9, 23 & 37.

## Additional acknowledgements

Page: 2-3 https://www.who.int/news-room/fact-sheets/detail/depression

With thanks to the Independence team: Shelley Baldry, Klaudia Sommer and Jackie Staines. Contributing Editor: Tracy Biram

Danielle Lobban

Cambridge, June 2022